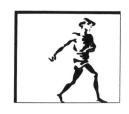

Frank and Christine Zane

ALSO BY FRANK AND CHRISTINE ZANE—
The Zane Way to a Beautiful Body

SUPER BODIES IN 12 WEEKS

Photography by JACK MITCHELL

SIMON AND SCHUSTER • NEW YORK

Copyright © 1981 by Frank and Christine Zane
All rights reserved
including the right of reproduction
in whole or in part in any form
Published by Simon and Schuster
A Division of Gulf & Western Corporation
Simon & Schuster Building
Rockefeller Center
1230 Avenue of the Americas
New York, New York 10020
SIMON AND SCHUSTER and colophon are trademarks of Simon & Schuster
Designed by Eve Metz
Manufactured in the United States of America

10 9 8 7 6 5 4 3 2 1

Library of Congress Cataloging in Publication Data

Zane, Frank.
    Frank and Christine Zane Super Bodies in 12 weeks.

    Includes index.
    1. Exercise. 2. Physical fitness. 3. Nutrition.
I. Zane, Christine. II. Title. III. Title: Super
Bodies in 12 weeks
RA781.Z36   613.7'1   81-14600
                                AACR2
ISBN 0-671-42077-1

ACKNOWLEDGMENTS

Special thanks to:
Dr. and Mrs. E. L. Hexberg, D.C., for their devotion
to the health and well-being of others
and to our parents
Josephine and Robert Harris
Laura and Adam Zane

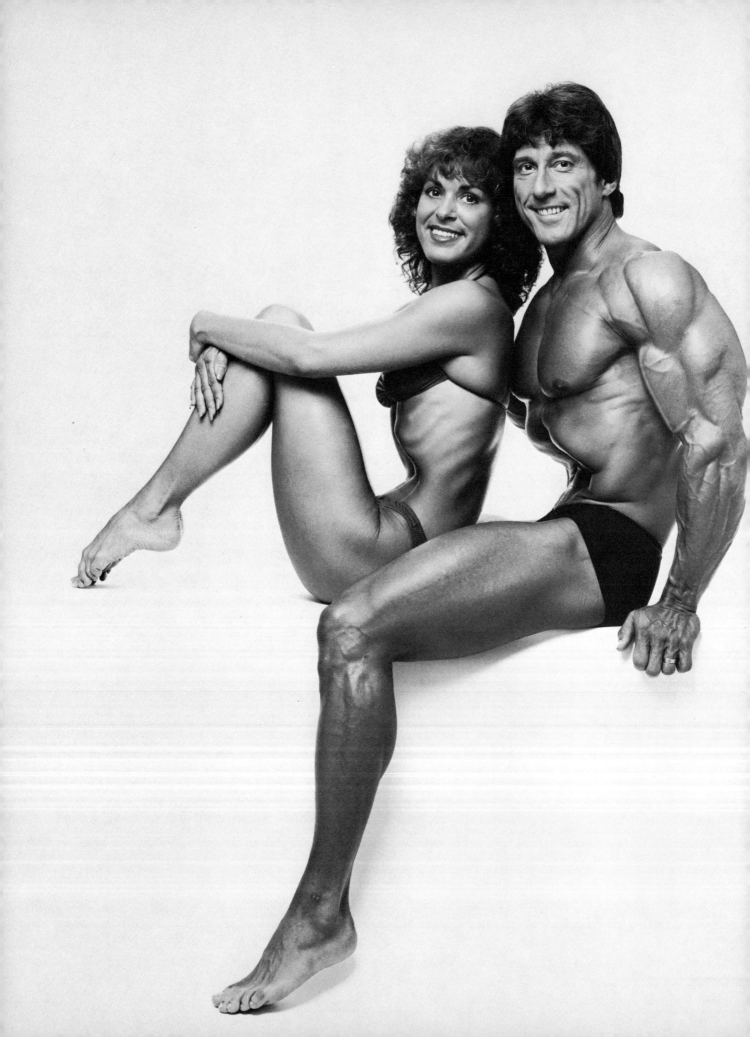

WE DEDICATE THIS BOOK TO EACH OTHER.

Contents

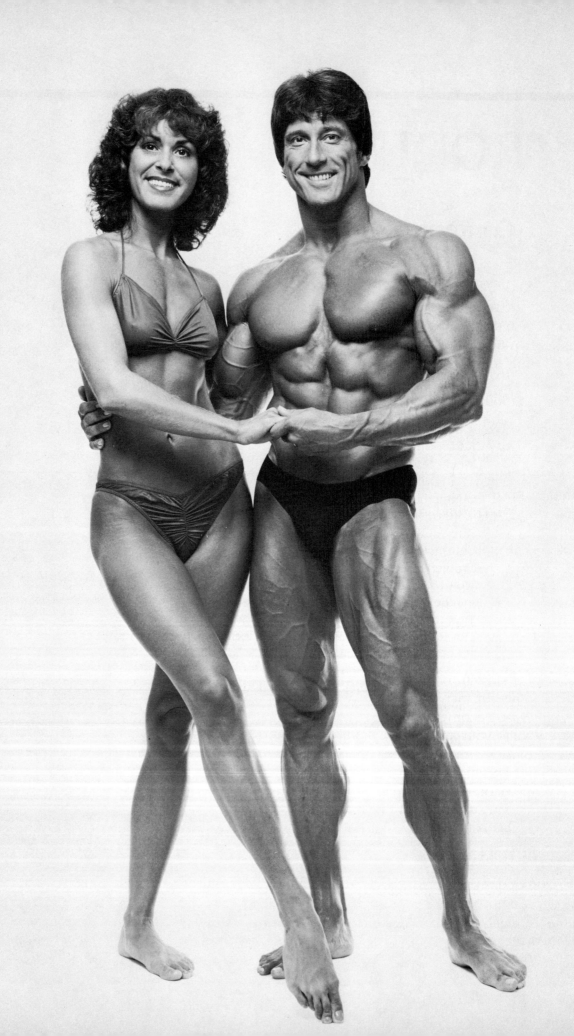

INTRODUCTION

THIS BOOK IS BASED ON our personal experience of combining rigorous exercise with a first-rate nutritional program. We have found the ideal length of time to allow oneself to reach peak physical condition is twelve weeks. Our book is a detailed day-by-day 12-week guide using a minimum amount of equipment, which combines weight training, stretching, aerobics, nutrition and body awareness in a program anyone can follow. You don't have to worry about what to do next because your entire program has been carefully planned. Since the intensity of the exercises increases gradually, stress is kept at a minimum and pleasure from seeing quick results at a maximum. The programs and exercises take you through a new world of sensations and stimulation; you will feel your body as you never have before.

Because nutrition is so important for developing a super body, we have devoted a special section of the book to that subject. Daily aerobic exercises with a gradual buildup of intensity are given to improve cardiovascular as well as muscular fitness. To develop body flexibility, stretching exercises accompany all weight-training movements and are practiced between each set. Flexibility is often neglected in weight-training routines, but in our book each muscle contraction is balanced with a strong stretch to the corresponding body area. We also give you techniques for increasing body awareness in the belief that the more aware you become of how your body looks, the more power you will have to alter your appearance in a positive way. Our mutual-assistance techniques enable both partners to strengthen their exercise relationship by giving each other positive reinforcement and support —and simultaneously experiencing that indescribable feeling of exhilaration that comes from getting in shape.

Physical Checkup

Before you begin your program, it is a good idea to see a physician and have a complete physical examination—to make sure there is nothing physically wrong with you. You should have a checkup at least once a year.

Assessing Your Physical Potential

Just because a woman trains with weights doesn't mean she'll become as muscular as a man. The truth is that she can lose body fat and tone muscles in selected areas in a relatively short time—and not have to worry about becoming too muscular. Women naturally have a higher percentage of body fat than men, so an appearance of firm shapeliness generally results from training. Also, because women have lower levels of testosterone, it is impossible for them to develop the same overall degree of muscularity as men. Because of this, men should be stronger than women in their upper bodies, but in the hips and legs women are proportionately stronger (probably because of the ability to bear children).

In general, both men and women should strive to develop well-proportioned bodies, with no one part built up at the expense of another: The upper body should not be too large or too small for the lower body.

Be realistic about your physical advantages and limitations. You cannot change your bone structure, but you can change the development and shape of the muscles. A person with wide hips cannot make the bone structure of this area any narrower, but he/she can make the hips appear smaller by increasing the size of the deltoids (shoulders) and upper back. Your metabolism or the rate at which your body burns food, may not be as good as you would like it to be, but you will find that with regular exercising it will improve and you will lose excess body fat.

Bodybuilding is the science of improving physical development, shaping muscles and reducing body fat through the practice of exercise and good nutrition. Your body will change as your mental image of it changes. To see these transformations, take color slides or photographs of yourself at different points in the program. Pictures are much more helpful than the scale or tape measure. Any camera will do, and you can project the 35-millimeter color slides life-size so that you can study them in great detail.

Resolve to make the most of your physical potential, whatever it may be.

Message to Teenagers

The early teens is a good time to start a regular exercising program. It is a time to learn how to improve and take care of your body and to use these good habits for the rest of your life. Frank was 14 when he started weight training and has been exercising ever since. You can build muscle and gain solid body weight if you are thin, or trim fat and improve the way you look and feel about yourself if you are overweight. You can get stronger for sports by following our methods and gain respect from your peers as they notice your physical improvement. As you develop your body, your self-confidence will increase and you'll have more energy to accomplish whatever you choose.

Start at the first level, the Basic Program. Follow the instructions right through Day 84. You'll be amazed at your progress.

Everyday Training

You will be doing weight training and aerobic exercises 6 days out of 7 each week. It is actually easier to exercise 6 days a week than 3 days a week when you are trying to get into your best condition. A schedule like this also helps reinforce the habit of regular exercise. You spend a shorter time exercising each day and you get the benefits of improved circulation, strength and physical vitality. The exercise sessions described in this book should take between 20 minutes and 1 hour and 15 minutes each day. You really don't need more training time than this to show great results, unless you are a competitive bodybuilder training for a contest. Even competitive bodybuilders, however, train as outlined in this book at certain times during the year.

Your 12-week program for a super body is organized into three 4-week phases. Weeks 1 through 4 (Days 1 through 28) constitute the Basic Program. You exercise 6 days a week, with a rest day on the seventh. On the first day and on alternate days thereafter, the muscles of the upper body are trained with weights and stretched (chest, shoulders, back and arms). On the second day and alternate days thereafter, the muscles of the lower body are trained (thighs, calves, waist). Therefore, the whole body is trained every 2 days, and each of the body parts is exercised three times a week.

The Intermediate Program is followed in Weeks 5 through 8 (Days 29 through 56). It is also used 6 days a week with a rest on the seventh day. Every 3 days the program is repeated. On the first and the fourth day of each week the pulling muscles are weight-trained and stretched (back, biceps, forearms); on the second and fifth days of each week the legs are trained (thighs and calves); on the third and the sixth days of each week the pushing muscles are worked (chest, shoulders, triceps). The waist is trained on every workout day 6 days each week. The whole body is trained every 3 days. Each body part is exercised twice a week, but more exercises and stretches are done for each body part than in the Basic Program.

The Advanced Program is performed in the same manner as the Intermediate Program, working each body part twice a week but doing still more exercises and stretches for each part of the body.

Choosing Your Level of Training

Each of these programs is divided into three levels of progression. Choose your level according to what your goals are and how much time you want to spend exercising each day. The levels differ in how many sets are done and in the number of repetitions performed during each set. Also, as you progress to each higher level, the stretches are held for a longer time. The first level is perfect for people who don't have a lot of time to exercise each day (20 to 30 minutes) but want to stay trim and well toned. One set of each weight-training exercise is immediately followed by a 10-second stretch. When your breathing returns to normal you go right to the next weight-training exercise, which is again immediately followed by a 10-second stretch. The emphasis in this first level of training is on performing all exercises correctly. The first level is a good one to choose if you haven't done much exercise prior to starting these programs.

The middle level is for those who want to increase the size and strength of their muscles. It emphasizes feeling the exercises in the exact areas intended. Each workout at this level takes about twice as long to complete as the first level. Each weight-training exercise is immediately followed by a 15-second stretch, then a short rest period to allow the breathing rate to return to normal. Then a second set of the same exercise is done again, immediately followed by the same 15-second stretch. After breathing returns to normal, you go on to the next weight-training exercise and stretch, doing 2 sets of each in the same manner. Always increase the amount of weight used at the middle level even if you have to do fewer repetitions. The middle level should be used by those who have had some prior experience with weight training, and can also be used by those who have just completed the 12-week program at the first level and wish to gain strength and develop a harder, firmer look to their bodies.

The top level is for people who have more time to exercise (at least 1 hour, 6 days a week) and want to get maximum results. As before, each weight-training exercise is followed by a stretching exercise, but this time the stretch is held for 20 seconds. Three sets of each weight-training exercise are followed by 3 stretches before moving on to the next weight-training exercise and stretch.

At the top level of training try to rest as little as possible between sets. Don't worry too much about increasing the weight on every set. Your main concern is moving through your workout without wasting time. This kind of training promotes excellent muscle tone and definition. The top level of training should be followed by those who either have had 6 months of prior weight-training experience or have just completed the 12-week program at the middle level.

Each of these levels is different from the others, and each succeeding one is progressively more difficult. Your body has a tendency to become accustomed to the exercises that you do for it. If you always follow the same program with the same intensity of exercise, you will eventually reach a "sticking point" where your progress comes to a near standstill. The key to successful exercising is to periodically vary your workouts and the way you do them. This way, as soon as your body starts adapting to what you are doing, you progressively intensify your program and avoid these unwanted sticking points. By following these programs as they are outlined at the first, middle and top levels you will be able to do just that.

Using This Book for Greater Progress

Your 12-week program is designed to be read one day at a time. But if you wish to read ahead a day to prepare yourself for the next day's program, feel free to do so. Following this program day by day helps you to concentrate on all the little details that ordinarily might be overlooked. In addition to the advice you receive each day on your total exercise program, the fine points of each weight-training exercise and stretch will be pointed out. Be sure to study these carefully; because how you do the exercise determines how you will shape and tone your body.

BASIC
PROGRAM

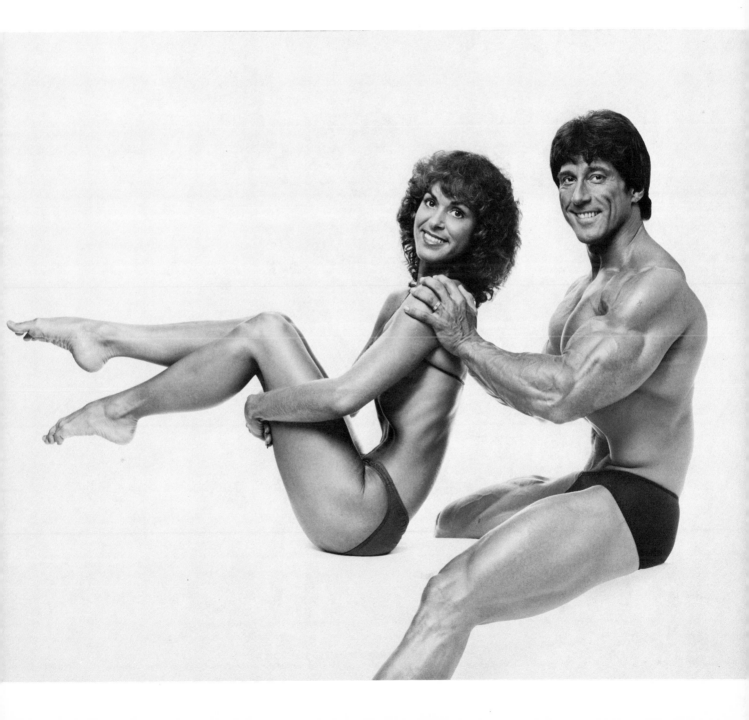

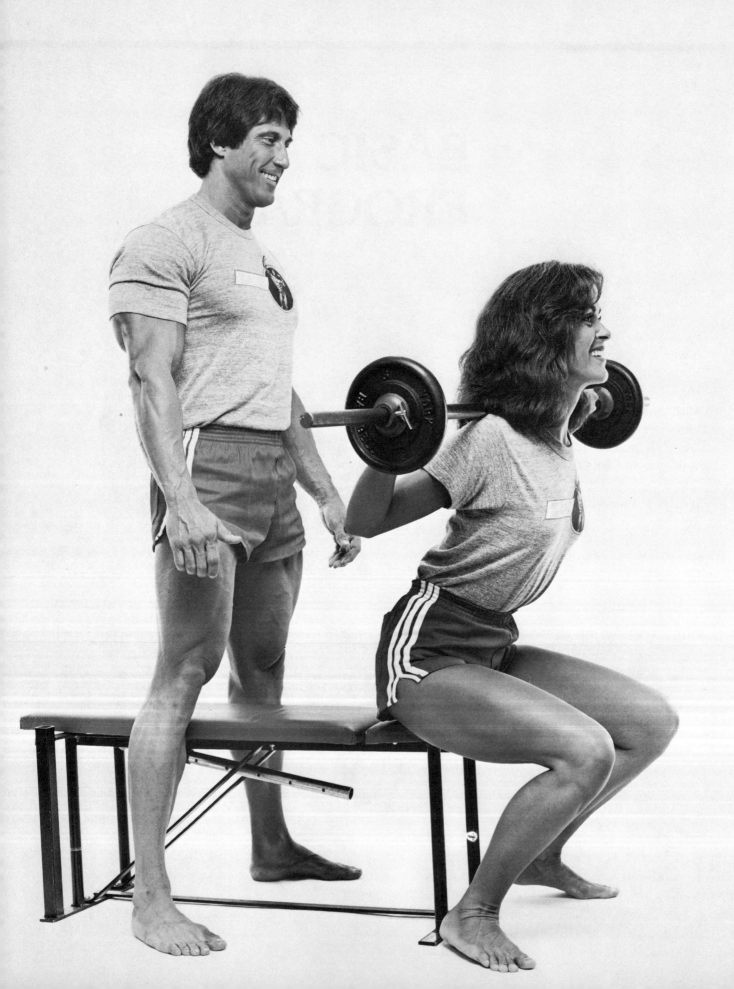

No matter what kind of shape you're in this Basic Program will be your starting point. During the next 4 weeks you will begin a bodybuilding split routine. You will divide your complete body program between 2 days: on Day 1 you will work the muscles of the upper body; on Day 2 you will work the muscles of the lower body. You will continue alternating your workouts in this manner. This will give you an opportunity to do more exercises per body part in relatively the same time as you would normally spend in the gym each day. By doing this, you will achieve results faster and more easily. Each day you are told exactly what to do: how to determine how much weight to use, and how many repetitions and sets to do.

The equipment that you will need to follow this program is minimal. A bench with an adjustable incline is preferred, but a flat bench will do as long as you have some way of elevating one end of it. Look for a sturdy bench, something like the one pictured in this section. You will also need a set of adjustable dumbbells to use with 5 to 35 pounds each; an adjustable barbell to use with 25 to 150 pounds total; a pair of ankle weights (2½ to 5 pounds each); a wooden pole or the end of a broomstick 5 feet long; a calf block or a step (the calf block we are shown using can be constructed out of 2-by-4 lumber and nails); a jump rope and a timer. Remember, the quality of your body development can often be determined by the quality of the equipment you have available, but high-quality equipment doesn't always mean expensive equipment. Make sure your equipment will stand up to use and abuse. It should be sturdy and safe. The equipment we have suggested is very versatile and can be worked with at home in a small space and stored in a closet when not in use.

Aerobic Exercises

Aerobic exercises should be done daily either each morning after rising or before your workout. When done properly, aerobic exercises will condition the heart, lungs and circulatory system, and will increase your level of endurance in daily activity, as well as in your weight training. This buildup takes place primarily as a result of increased amounts of oxygen being pumped quickly through your system.

For a "true" aerobic effect, however, the heart rate must remain at a level above normal for a period of at least 15 minutes. With practice, this is not difficult to achieve with forms of exercise such as jogging or fast walking. The aerobic exercises given here are too difficult for most people to do for extended periods. These exercises work more muscles of the body than jogging or fast walking, but do not provide as much of an aerobic effect because they are not continued for a long enough time. We have found, however, that even as little as a few minutes a day of our aerobic exercises, when combined with our weight-training and stretching exercise programs, will help you experience many of the same benefits of "true" aerobic exercise. Keeping your rest periods down and your heart rate up during your workouts also gives you many of the aerobic benefits.

If you have been jogging or doing fast walking, or if you wish to do so in conjunction with your weight training, follow the daily aerobic exercises that we describe and then go out for your walk or jog. If you're just starting, here's a good schedule:

Jogging (slow running)—6 days a week

    Week 1—½ mile in 5 minutes
    Week 2—¾ mile in 7½ minutes
    Week 3—1 mile in 10 minutes
    Week 4—1¼ miles in 12½ minutes
    Week 5—1½ miles in 15 minutes

If you wish to spend more than 15 minutes jogging, then continue adding ¼ mile each week. Be sure to warm up with stretching exercises like the Wall Lean (page 96), Forward Stretch (page 47), One-Leg-up Stretch (page 123), and Lunge on Step (page 46) for a few minutes before you run.

If you have sore knees or trouble with sore tibialis (shin splints), you may wish to do fast walking 6 days a week. Your schedule should be:

    Week 1—1 mile in 20 minutes
    Week 2—1½ miles in 30 minutes
    Week 3—2 miles in 40 minutes
    Week 4—2½ miles in 50 minutes
    Week 5—3 miles in 60 minutes

Anaerobic Exercises

Weight training is the major focus of this program. It is a form of anaerobic exercise.

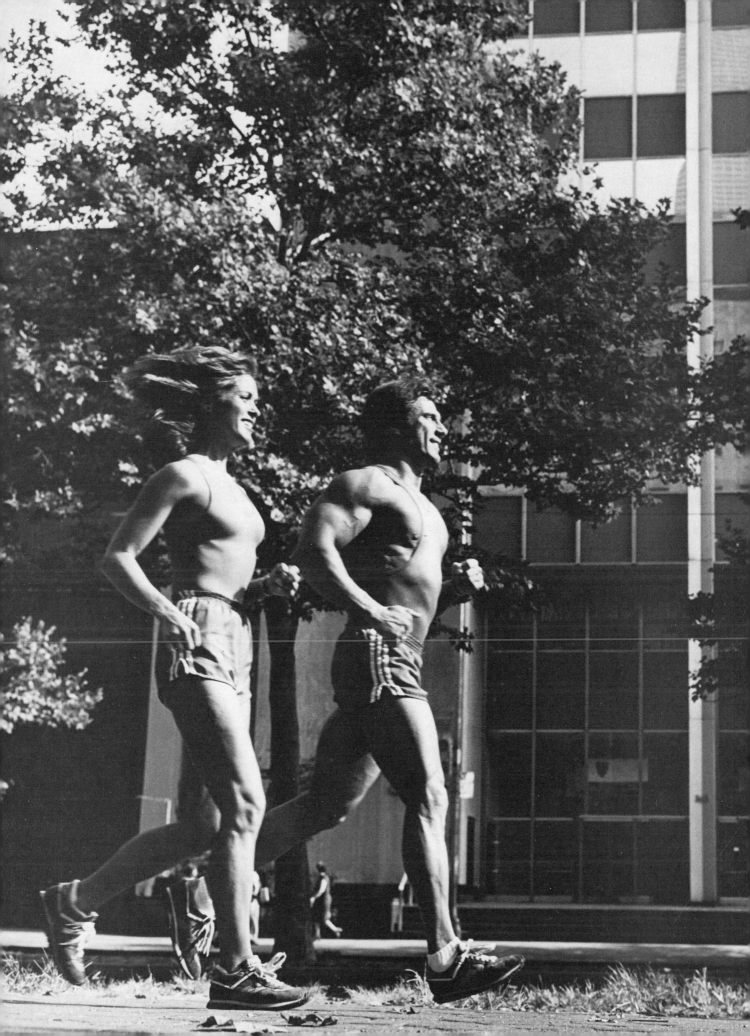

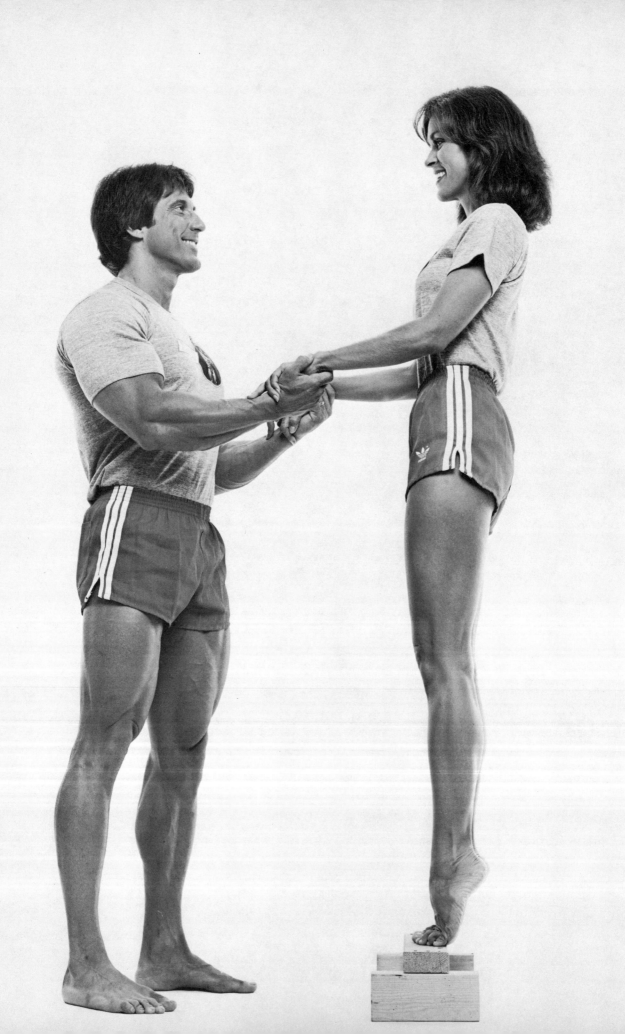

Weight-training exercises demand that your body use a lot of oxygen in a short time. At the end of your set of repetitions you create an oxygen debt that must be paid quickly. This is why you need time, usually 1 to 3 minutes, depending on the intensity of the anaerobic exercise, to rest between sets.

The aerobic exercises described in this book will give you more endurance and make it easier for you to spend less time resting between sets. Keep rest periods at a minimum for a trimmer, well-toned body.

Stretching

Along with the weight-training anaerobic exercises, you will be doing various stretching movements that will help to relax the muscles and to counter the flexing movement in the exercise. Stretching exercises are also very helpful in warming up and relieving tension in a muscle before it is worked. You will notice that there is not a stretch for every weight-training movement. Many weight-training exercises are very effective stretching movements as well. In these exercises you will be told when to get the maximum stretch.

Diet and Nutrition

The way in which you eat and care for your body is a crucial aspect of getting and staying in shape. Your progress can be slowed or diverted by bad nutrition or unhealthful habits. Each week we will give you some appropriate diet tips that we have found work extremely well for us. We will make suggestions for you to follow in the choice and preparation of your food which will help you reach your goal rapidly, but in a gradual and safe manner. We will assist you in becoming aware of your eating habits. You will be amazed at the results!

Mutual-Assistance Techniques

Each week we will give you advice on how to derive the most benefit from training with a partner. We call this part of the program "mutual-assistance techniques," because in these sections we explain how you can help each other have a better workout and move successfully toward reaching your goal.

Here is some bodybuilding vocabulary that you'll need to know:

AEROBIC—Exercises that condition the heart, lungs and circulatory systems.
ANAEROBIC—Exercises (usually weight training) that develop and tone muscles.

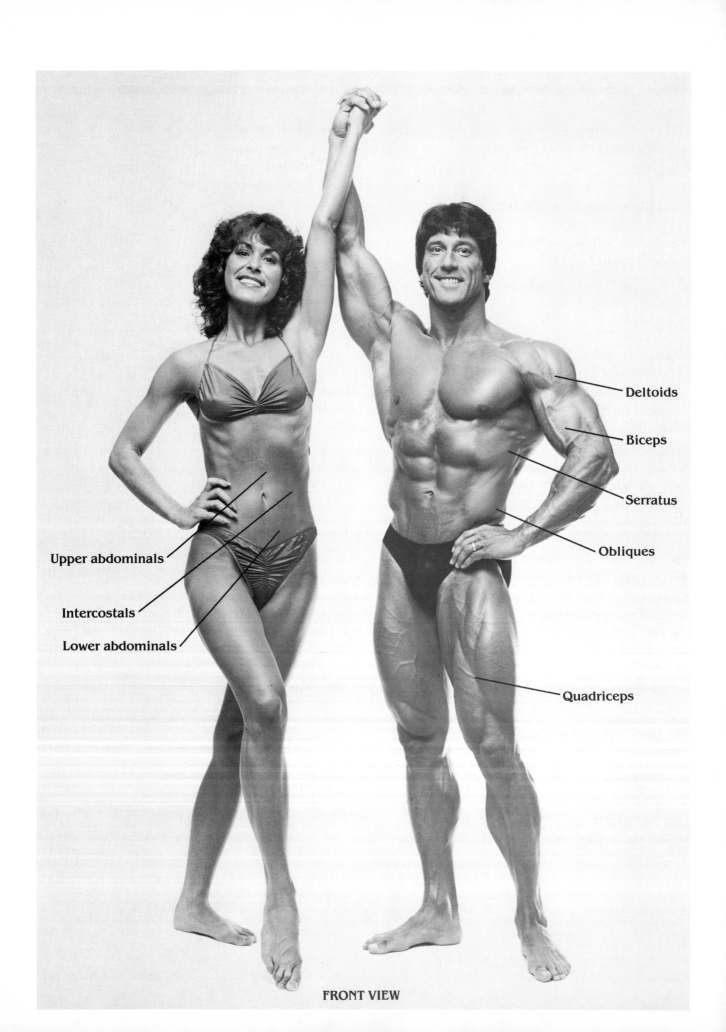

Deltoids

Biceps

Serratus

Obliques

Upper abdominals

Intercostals

Lower abdominals

Quadriceps

FRONT VIEW

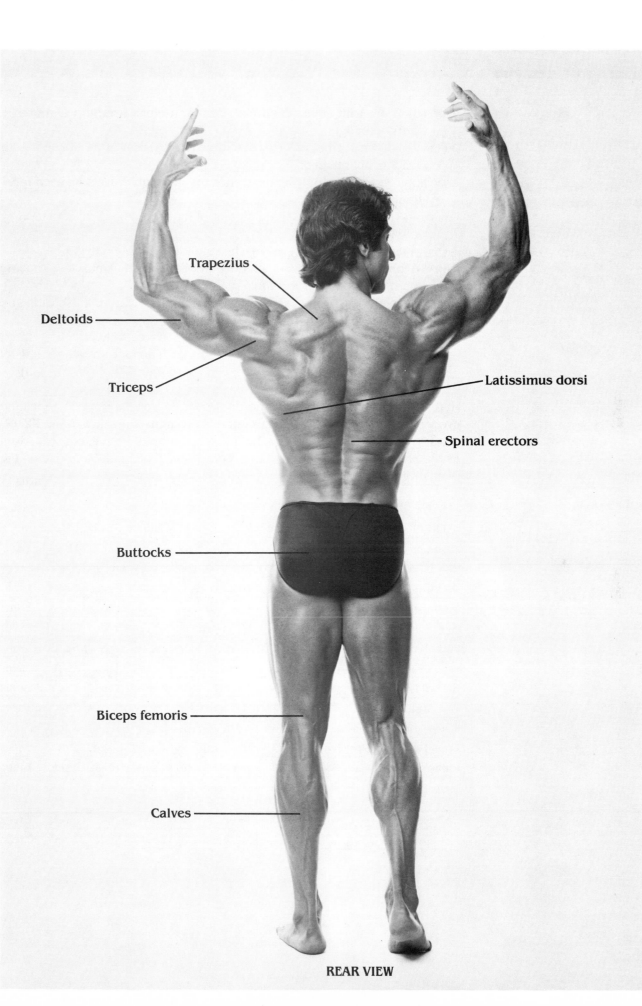

Trapezius

Deltoids

Triceps

Latissimus dorsi

Spinal erectors

Buttocks

Biceps femoris

Calves

REAR VIEW

BARBELL—A bar with adjustable weights at both ends, used in weight-resistance training.

DUMBBELL—A weight held in each hand which consists of a short bar with weights at both ends.

GROOVE—The pathway of least resistance that a weight travels on each repetition.

PEAKING—The science of reaching a point of maximum physical condition by following a plan.

PRESS—Pushing a weight overhead while standing, sitting or lying.

PUMP—A physical sensation of blood pumping into the muscles, causing them to temporarily expand.

REPS (or repetitions)—One complete movement from start to finish within an exercise.

SETS—A specified number of repetitions done consecutively.

STICKING POINT—The place where your progress comes to a near standstill necessitating a change in the exercise program.

Here are the exercises you will be doing starting on Day 1, and repeating every other day for the first 4 weeks of this program (Days 1, 3, 5, 8, 10, 12, 15, 17, 19, 22, 24 and 26). For the full description of each exercise, as well as the photos showing start and finish positions, look up the exercise on the page given in the chart below.

EXERCISE	Page	First Level	Middle Level	Top Level
Push-ups (warm-up)	27	1 set, 10 reps	1 set, 10 reps	1 set, 10 reps
Bench Press	28	1 set, 10 reps	2 sets, 8 reps	3 sets, 12 reps
Doorway Stretch	29	10 seconds	2 sets, 15 sec	3 sets, 20 sec
Dumbbell Pullover	30	1 set, 10 reps	2 sets, 8 reps	3 sets, 12 reps
Overhead Stretch	31	10 seconds	2 sets, 15 sec	3 sets, 20 sec
Press Behind Neck	32	1 set, 10 reps	2 sets, 8 reps	3 sets, 12 reps
One-Arm Shoulder Stretch	33	10 seconds	2 sets, 15 sec	3 sets, 20 sec
Barbell Row	34	1 set, 10 reps	2 sets, 8 reps	3 sets, 12 reps
One-Arm Lat Stretch	35	10 seconds	2 sets, 15 sec	3 sets, 20 sec
Close-Grip Bench Press	36	1 set, 10 reps	2 sets, 8 reps	3 sets, 12 reps
Arms-Backward Stretch	37	10 seconds	2 sets, 15 sec	3 sets, 20 sec
Barbell Curl	38	1 set, 10 reps	2 sets, 8 reps	3 sets, 12 reps
Arms-Backward Stretch with Pronation	39	10 seconds	2 sets, 15 sec	3 sets, 20 sec
Reverse Curl	40	1 set, 10 reps	2 sets, 8 reps	3 sets, 12 reps
Fist Curl, Wrist Down	41	10 seconds	2 sets, 15 sec	3 sets, 20 reps

PUSH-UPS

Lie face down on the floor with your hands beside your shoulders, palms down, fingers forward. Rest your feet on the toes only. Keep your body straight, as you push with your hands and arms until your elbows are straight. Lower yourself slowly until almost touching the floor. Exhale when you start the exercise (pushing up) and inhale as you lower yourself to the floor. Push-ups are good to warm up with before doing Bench Press. Both exercises work the same areas. In order to avoid muscle pulls and injuries, it is essential always to do some type of warm-up exercise before using weights. As you do each push-up you will feel the blood circulating in the chest, shoulders (especially the front part of the shoulders) and triceps (backs of arms). If 10 reps of regular push-ups are too difficult for you, then do push-ups while up on your knees. These are done in the same manner as regular push-ups but using the knees instead of the feet as a pivot point. See exercise photo.

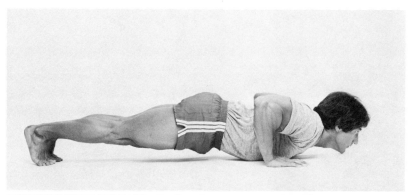

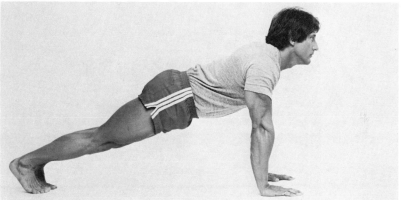

Push-ups (regular)

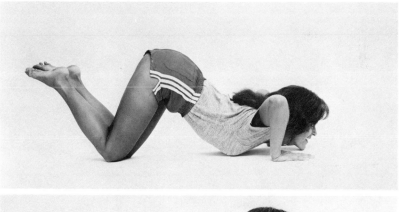

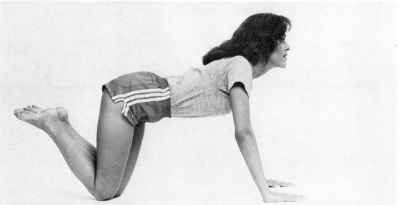

Push-ups (on knees)

27

BENCH PRESS

First level: 1 set, 10 reps
Middle level: 2 sets, 8 reps
Top level: 3 sets, 12 reps

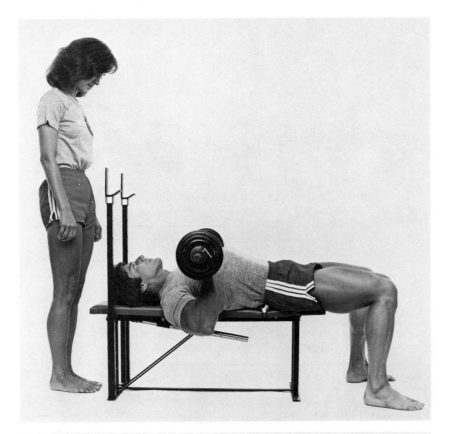

Lie on your back on a flat bench. Either place your feet on the floor to each side, or place them on the bench with your knees bent. Hold the barbell with hands about shoulder width apart. Inhale and slowly lower the bar to your chest (nipple level). Exhale as you push the barbell straight up until your elbows are straight. Bench Press is an excellent exercise for the chest, shoulders and triceps. After doing your designated number of repetitions with the correctly chosen weight, you will feel an expanding sensation in the pectoral (chest) muscles and in the front part of your deltoids (shoulder) and triceps. This is called the "pump." The expanded sensation is caused by blood rushing to aid the exercising muscles, which results in a feeling of firmness and strength. You should keep this feeling throughout your whole workout as you do the exercises that work each part of the body. Not only will your muscle tone improve by working for a pump but so will your circulation.

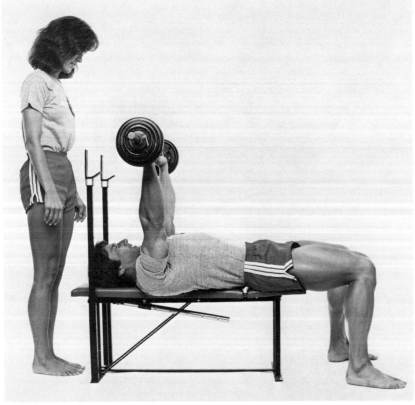

Always do the stretch immediately after completing the weight-training movement.

DOORWAY STRETCH

First level: 1 set, 10 sec
Middle level: 2 sets, 15 sec
Top level: 3 sets, 20 sec

Position your fists on the back of both sides of a doorway at hip level. Allow your body to lean slightly forward until your shoulders and chest feel the stretch. Hold this position for the designated time and then relax. This is an excellent stretch to do after chest exercises because it increases the effectiveness of the previous weight-training movements by promoting better blood circulation in this area, thus improving the development of the chest and front deltoids.

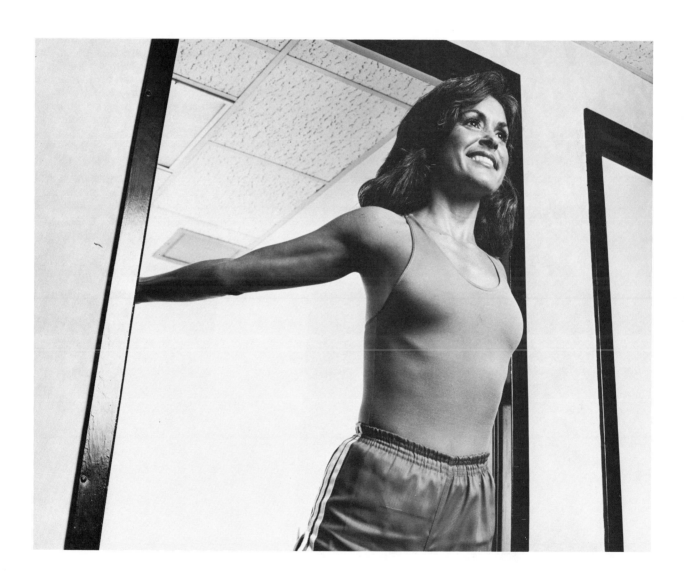

DUMBBELL PULLOVER

First level: 1 set, 10 reps
Middle level: 2 sets, 8 reps
Top level: 3 sets, 12 reps

Position yourself across a flat bench with your shoulders resting on the bench and your head hanging down over one side. Extend your legs straight together out the other side. Have your partner hand you the dumbbell, or reach back to the floor and lift it by holding it with both hands on one of the plates and thumbs around the dumbbell bar. Begin with the dumbbell over your forehead. Inhale and slowly lower the dumbbell until close to the floor behind you. Stretch and arch your back and rib cage. Exhale and bring the dumbbell back over your forehead. Keep your elbows slightly bent. This exercise lifts the rib cage and improves posture. It also works the serratus (the saw-toothed, jagged muscle formation approximately 6 inches below the armpit) and the rear part of the triceps muscle as well. You should experience a stretching, pulling feeling as you do each repetition.

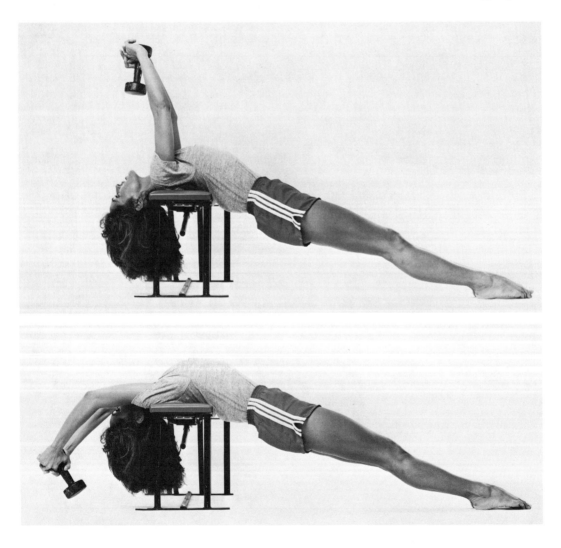

OVERHEAD STRETCH

First level: 1 set, 10 sec
Middle level: 2 sets, 15 sec
Top level: 3 sets, 20 sec

Do this exercise immediately after Pull-overs. Standing, clasp your hands together and turn them out as you stretch the palms of your hands upward. Stretch until you feel it down to the base of your spine. Hold the stretch for the designated time and then relax. You will feel the shoulder muscles working as well as the serratus and arm muscles stretching.

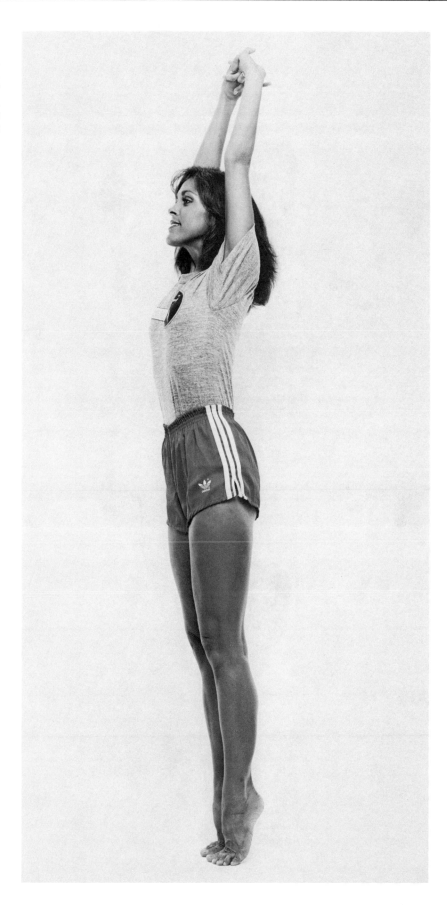

PRESS BEHIND NECK

First level: 1 set, 10 reps
Middle level: 2 sets, 8 reps
Top level: 3 sets, 12 reps

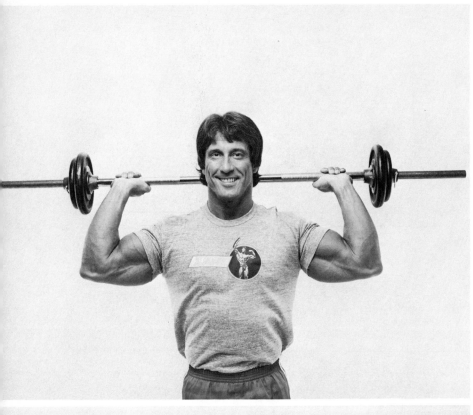

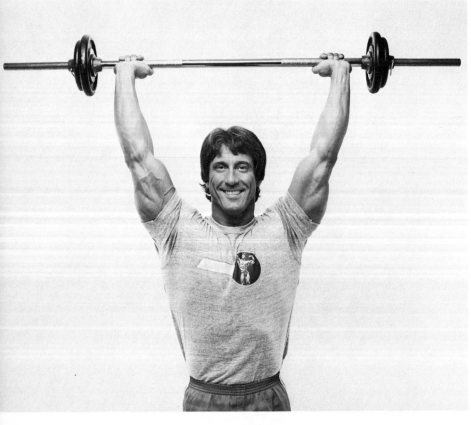

Stand erect or sit on the edge of a bench with a barbell resting across your shoulders, behind your neck. Hold the bar just outside each shoulder. Exhale as you press the barbell overhead until your elbows are straight. Move your head only slightly forward so that the bar doesn't hit your head. Inhale and lower the bar back to your shoulders. When the arms and elbows are held back as far as possible, this exercise directly works the front and side portions of the shoulder muscles (deltoids) as well as the rear deltoid. Your deltoids will feel pumped and expanded and your shoulders will appear wider after the set is completed.

ONE-ARM SHOULDER STRETCH

First level: 1 set, 10 sec
Middle level: 2 sets, 15 sec
Top level: 3 sets, 20 sec

Raise one arm until it is straight overhead and your elbow is very close to your head and back. Lower this hand until you can touch your upper back, keeping your elbow pressed against your head. Hold this position. Take your opposite hand and pull gently on the back of the stretched arm until you feel the stretch. Hold this position for the designated time. Relax and repeat with the other arm. This stretch loosens up the top of the shoulders and stretches the triceps as well. If one shoulder feels tighter than the other, repeat another 10-second stretch to loosen the tight shoulder.

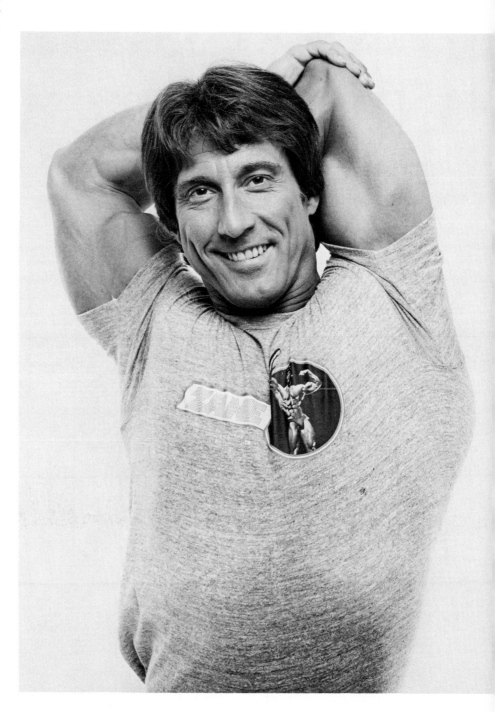

BARBELL ROW

First level: 1 set, 10 reps
Middle level: 2 sets, 8 reps
Top level: 3 sets, 12 reps

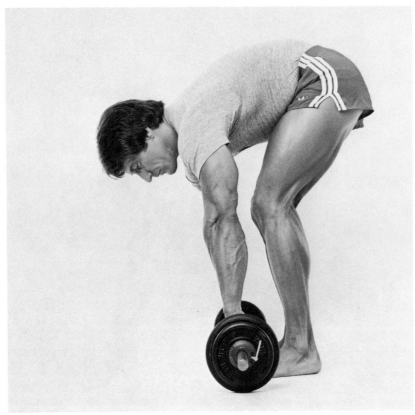

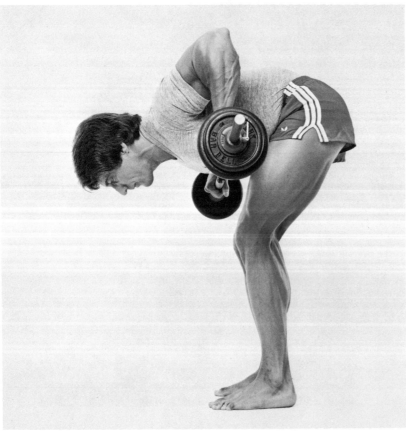

Standing with your feet less than shoulder-width distance apart (you may wish to stand on a block for a better stretch), bend forward at the waist and bend your knees. Your stomach should touch your thighs in this position. Let your hands go straight down, stretching as much as possible, and grasp the barbell at shoulder width (or with a slightly wider grip). Pull the barbell up to your chest, keeping your elbows out to each side. Touch the barbell just below the nipples and slowly lower it to the fullest stretching extension. Repeat without moving your torso from the initial position, keeping your back parallel to the floor at all times. Barbell Row is probably the best overall back exercise when done this way. You'll feel this exercise mainly in the latissimus dorsi muscles or the "lats"—the V-shaped muscles of the back. It is important to stretch down as far as possible so that you can feel the pump in the lower lats and develop this area.

ONE-ARM LAT STRETCH

First level: 1 set, 10 sec
Middle level: 2 sets, 15 sec
Top level: 3 sets, 20 sec

For this stretch, stand at a 45-degree angle to a vertical bar. Grasp the bar at hip level with the hand farthest from the bar, and bend at the waist with your knees bent. Pull away from the bar, stretching your back down to your waist. Repeat on the opposite side. You will feel the stretch from the base of each armpit down to the sides of the waist and possibly into the hip.

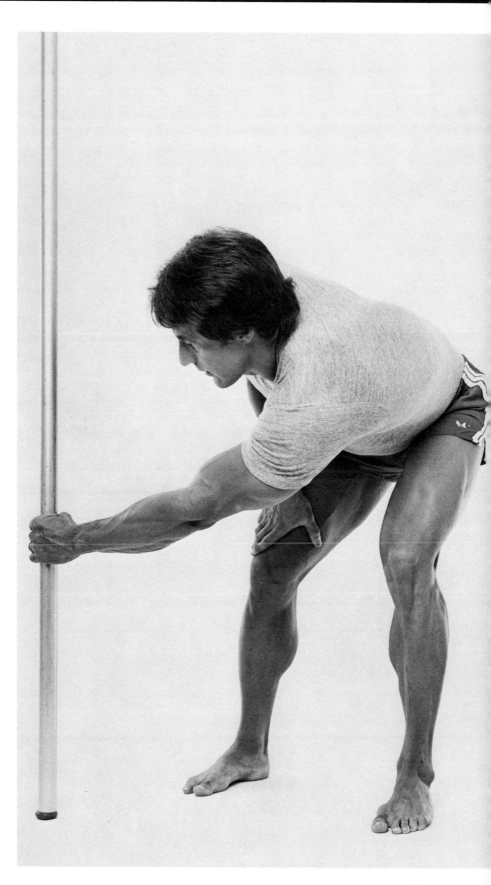

35

CLOSE-GRIP BENCH PRESS

First level: 1 set, 10 reps
Middle level: 2 sets, 8 reps
Top level: 3 sets, 12 reps

Lie on a flat bench with your feet resting flat on the floor on either side. Or bend your knees and rest your feet on the end of the bench. Hold the barbell over your chest, at nipple level, with the hands about 6 to 12 inches apart. Inhale and slowly lower the bar to your chest, keeping your elbows out to each side. Exhale and push the bar up until your arms are straight again. Tense the triceps as the arms straighten out and repeat. This exercise works the outer, lateral triceps.

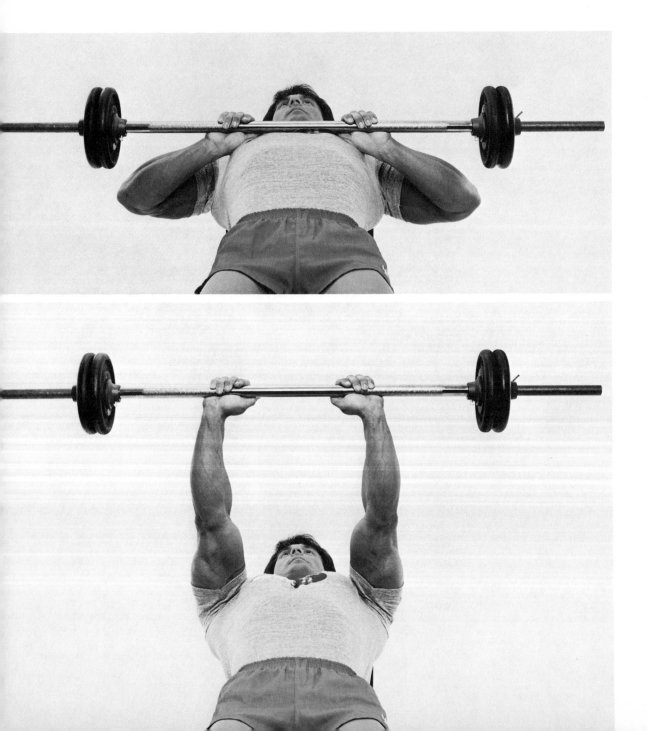

ARMS-BACKWARD STRETCH

First level: 1 set, 10 sec
Middle level: 2 sets, 15 sec
Top level: 3 sets, 20 sec

Stand erect with your arms down at each side. Turn your hands so the palms face backward. Bend your upper body slightly forward from the waist and push your hands back, keeping your elbows straight until you feel a stretch in the rear part of the upper arms and shoulders. Hold this position for the designated time, then relax. This stretch brings more blood into the triceps area and loosens the rear part of the shoulders. It is very good to do following any tricep exercise. Be sure to keep palms facing backward and you will feel an expanding and stretching sensation in the horseshoe-shaped tricep muscles.

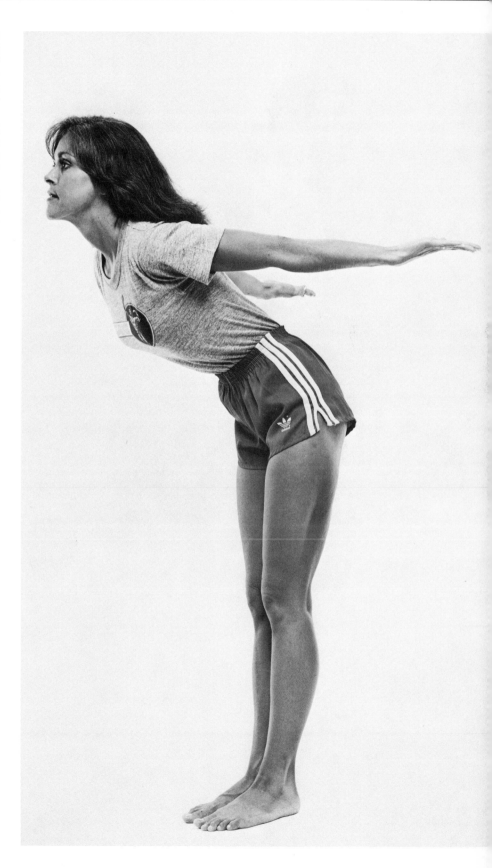

BARBELL CURL

First level: 1 set, 10 reps
Middle level: 2 sets, 8 reps
Top level: 3 sets, 12 reps

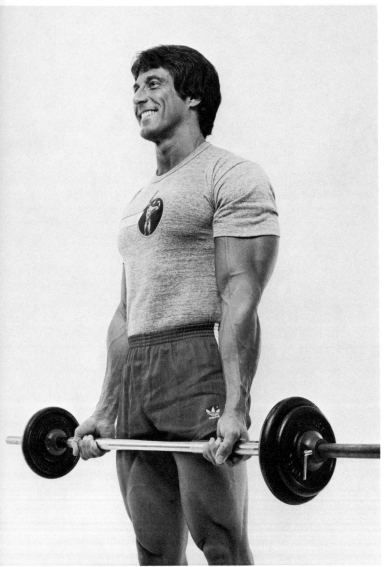

Standing, grasp a barbell with both hands using an underhand grip, and hold your arms straight down to each side. Your hands should rest close to the outside of each thigh. Keep your elbows in tight to your sides, inhale and curl the barbell in an arc upward until it touches your chin, keeping your wrists straight. Tense your biceps at this top position and then slowly lower the barbell as you exhale, returning to the starting position with your arms straight. Repeat for the designated number of repetitions. This exercise shapes and strengthens the bicep muscles. You'll feel the pump in the front part of your arm.

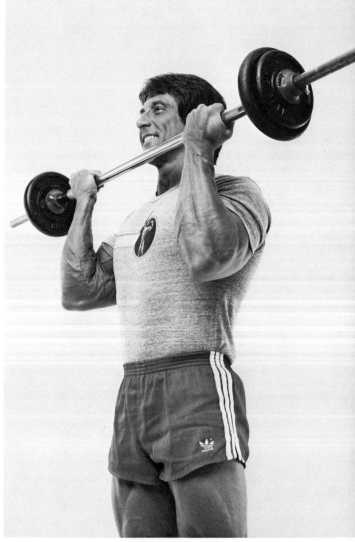

ARMS-BACKWARD STRETCH
WITH PRONATION

First level: 1 set, 10 sec
Middle level: 2 sets, 15 sec
Top level: 3 sets, 20 sec

Standing with your arms down to each side, turn your palms so that they face backward. Bend your upper body forward as you push your hands back, keeping your arms straight until you feel the stretch. In this position, pronate or turn the thumb side of your hands outward a little more and hold for the designated time. Then relax. This stretch should be done immediately after bicep work because it further stimulates this area. You will feel the stretch in the outer portion of the biceps.

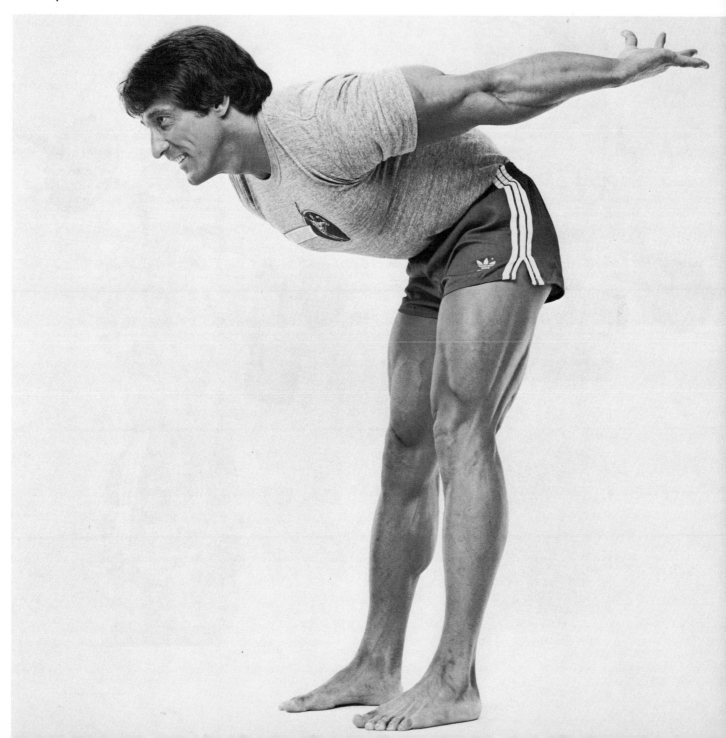

REVERSE CURL

First level: 1 set, 10 reps
Middle level: 2 sets, 8 reps
Top level: 3 sets, 12 reps

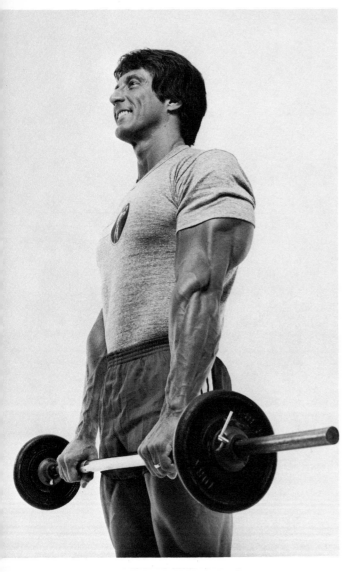

Standing, grip the barbell with an overhand grip and hold your arms down to each side. Your hands should be just outside of each thigh. Keep your wrists straight and your elbows in tight to each side as you inhale and curl the bar up in an arc until it touches your chin. Exhale as you slowly lower the barbell until your arms are straight again. Repeat for the designated number of times. This exercise strengthens the grip and develops the muscles of the forearms. Squeeze the bar and feel the forearms expanding and strengthening as you do each rep.

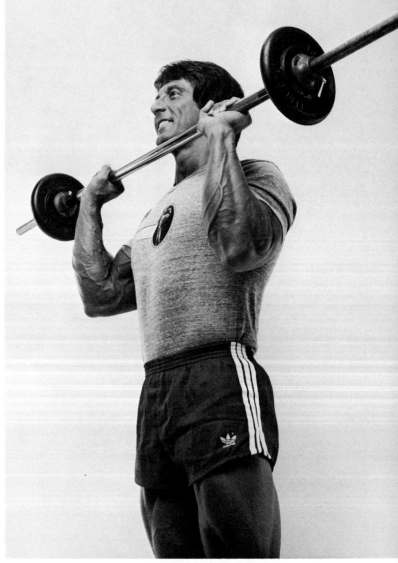

40

FIST CURL, WRIST DOWN

First level: 1 set, 10 sec
Middle level: 2 sets, 15 sec
Top level: 3 sets, 20 sec

This is a stretching movement that should be done along with forearm exercises. You will feel the stretch in the top of the forearm. It is done by holding the arms straight out in front of you, palms down and making a fist. Turn each fist downward by bending your wrist and holding this position for the designated amount of time.

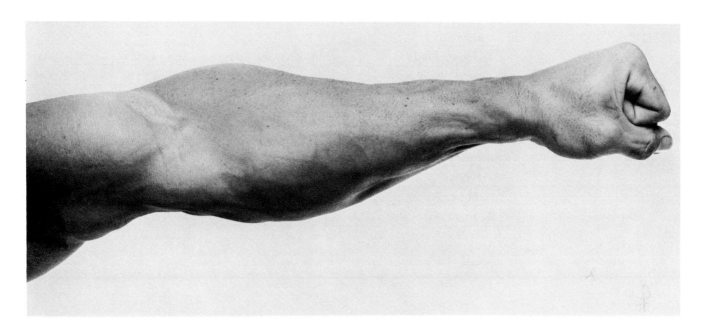

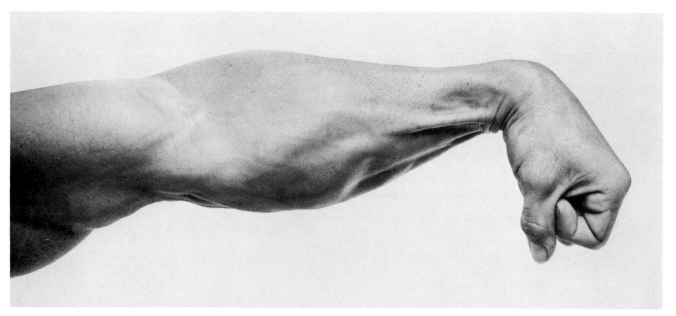

41

Here is the second part of your Basic Program. It completes your 2-day cycle in which you will have worked all the muscles of the body over a 2-day period. Follow this program on Days 2, 4, 6, 9, 11, 13, 16, 18, 20, 23, 25 and 27. For the full descriptions of each weight-training exercise and stretch, along with the start and finish position photos, look up the exercise on the page number given in the chart which follows.

EXERCISE	Page	First Level	Middle Level	Top Level
One-Leg Top Extension (warm-up)	43	1 set, 20 reps	1 set, 20 reps	1 set, 20 reps
Half Squat	44	1 set, 10 reps	2 sets, 8 reps	3 sets, 12 reps
Lunge with Back Foot on Bench	45	10 seconds	2 sets, 15 sec	3 sets, 20 sec
Lunge on Step	46	1 set, 10 reps	2 sets, 8 reps	3 sets, 12 reps
Forward Stretch	47	10 seconds	2 sets, 15 sec	3 sets, 20 sec
Donkey Calf Raise	48	1 set, 20 reps	2 sets, 15 reps	3 sets, 25 reps
One-Leg Calf Stretch	49	10 seconds	2 sets, 15 sec	3 sets, 20 sec
Free-Standing Calf Raise	50	1 set, 20 reps	2 sets, 15 reps	3 sets, 25 reps
Two-Leg Calf Stretch	51	10 seconds	2 sets, 15 sec	3 sets, 20 sec
Flat Knee-in	52	1 set, 20 reps	2 sets, 25 reps	3 sets, 30 reps
Bent-Leg Partial Sit-up	53	1 set, 20 reps	2 sets, 25 reps	3 sets, 30 reps
Seated Twist	54	1 set, 20 reps	2 sets, 25 reps	3 sets, 30 reps

ONE-LEG TOP EXTENSION

All levels: 1 set, 20 reps

Sit in a chair or on the edge of a sturdy table or high bench so that your legs dangle over the side. You may use a leg-extension table if you have access to one. One leg at a time, extend the foot in a flexed position until the entire leg is straight. Bring this leg back halfway and extend it again. Hold the leg for a moment at the full extension. Repeat these partial movements for all repetitions. Do the same for the other leg. Be sure to do each repetition slowly. This exercise warms up and strengthens the knee and the muscles directly above the knee (quadriceps). It is always a good idea to start all thigh-exercise programs with this exercise. It is especially good to do before any kind of squatting movements and is very effective in rehabilitating injured knees. When doing the first few repetitions, don't tense your thigh too hard. Instead increase the tension as you do each succeeding repetition.

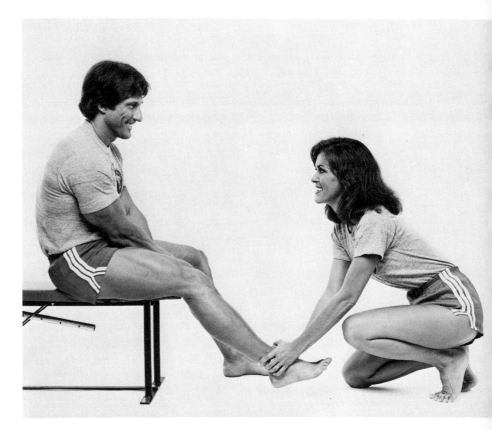

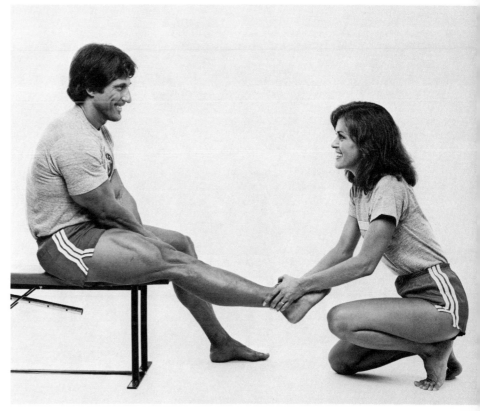

HALF SQUAT

First level: 1 set, 10 reps
Middle level: 2 sets, 8 reps
Top level: 3 sets, 12 reps

With your feet facing forward, straddle a bench with a barbell resting across your shoulders. Slowly descend to the bench, inhaling, and keeping your back erect. When you touch the bench, begin your ascent, exhaling as you come up until you are standing erect again. Do not sit on the bench. This exercise firms the buttocks and develops the entire thigh—especially the muscles of the upper thigh. You will feel the pump in the frontal, upper thigh muscles.

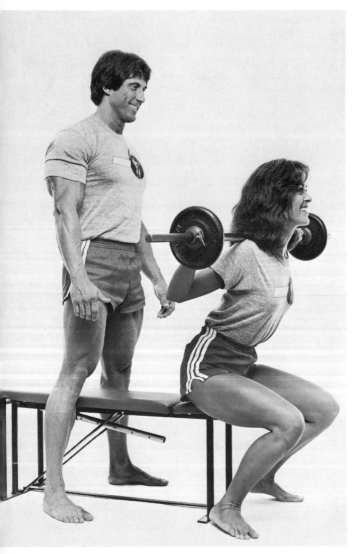
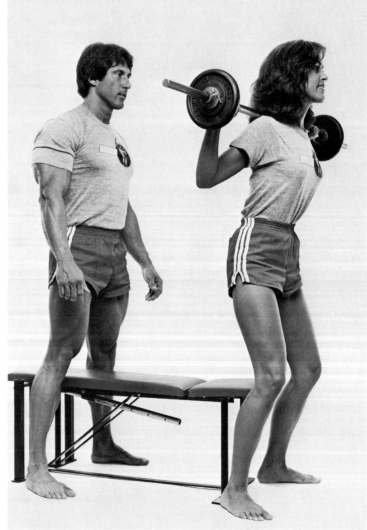

44

LUNGE WITH BACK FOOT ON BENCH

First level: 1 set, 10 sec
Middle level: 2 sets, 15 sec
Top level: 3 sets, 20 sec

This is a very effective stretching exercise for the frontal thigh. Stand a few feet in front of a bench, facing away from it. Place one foot back and on the bench with the sole of the foot facing upward. Lunge forward on the leg that is on the floor, bending the knee until you feel the stretching in the front of the opposite thigh. Hold this stretch for the designated time, and then relax and repeat with the other leg.

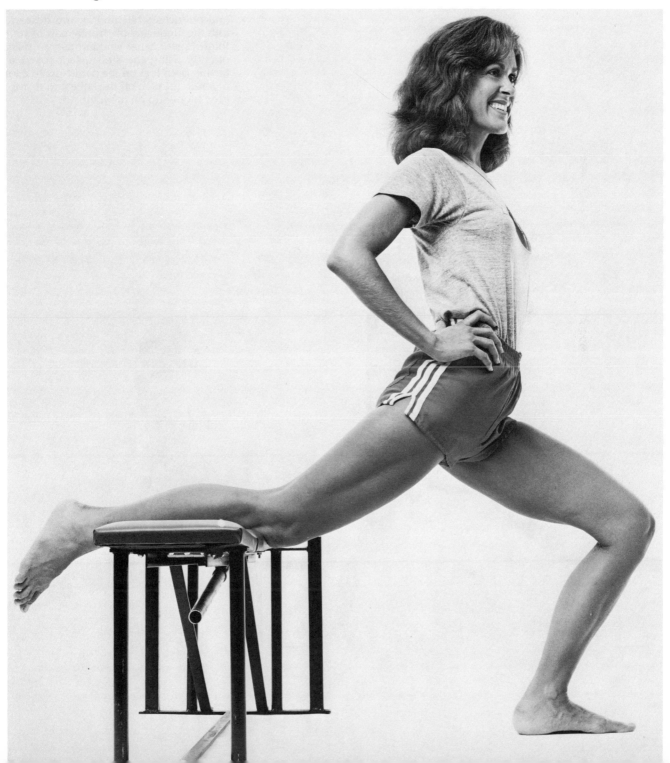

LUNGE ON STEP

First level: 1 set, 10 reps
Middle level: 2 sets, 8 reps
Top level: 3 sets, 12 reps

Holding a dumbbell in each hand, place one foot on a bench or the second or third step of a staircase, and extend the other leg back so that the toes only are resting on the floor. Inhale as you bend the raised leg and lunge toward the step, keeping your back straight. Exhale as you slowly push with the raised leg until it is straight again. Repeat for the designated number of repetitions and then change your position to work the opposite leg. You should feel the back of your thighs and buttocks stretching as you descend into the lunge and the frontal part of your thigh (quadriceps) working as you push out. By using the step (as opposed to having both feet on the same level), a lot of strain is taken off the knee and distributed higher up on the thigh.

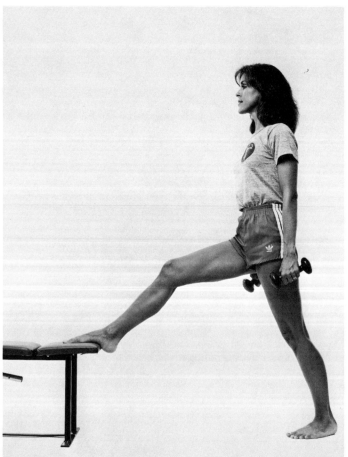
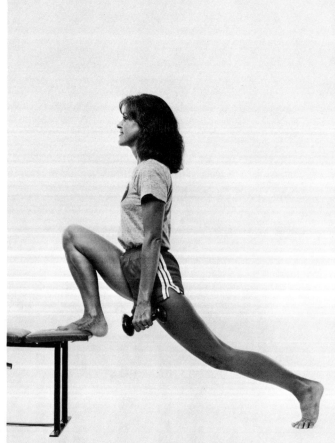

FORWARD STRETCH

First level: 1 set, 10 sec
Middle level: 2 sets, 15 sec
Top level: 3 sets, 20 sec

Standing with your feet shoulder distance apart, knees straight (if you have lower-back problems, keep your knees slightly bent) and arms at your sides, inhale as you lift both arms straight overhead. Exhale and keep your arms straight as you bend forward and touch your toes, very slowly. Hold this position for the designated time and then return to the erect position and relax. Remember not to bounce, and to stretch as close to the floor as possible. Don't worry if you can't make it all the way to the lowest position at first. Your flexibility will improve as you continue to do this exercise. This stretch loosens the backs of the thighs (leg biceps) and the lower-back or spinal-erector muscles. You'll feel these areas stretching as you hold in the low position.

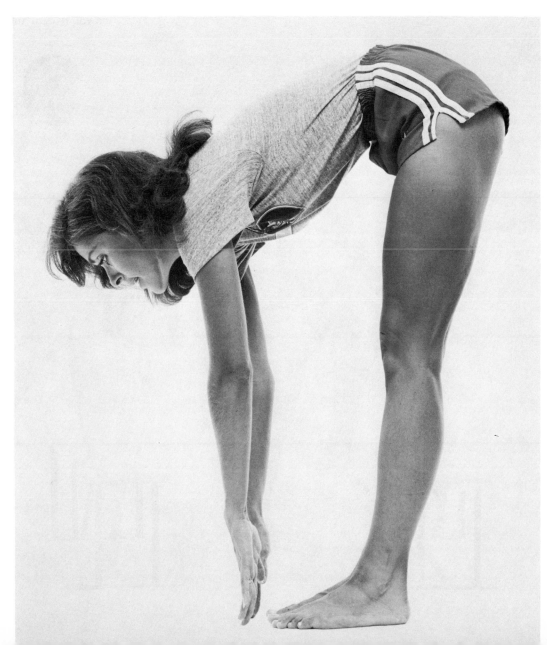

DONKEY CALF RAISE

First level: 1 set, 20 reps
Middle level: 2 sets, 15 reps
Top level: 3 sets, 25 reps

Place your feet on the calf block (with about one-third of the front part of your foot resting on the block) and bend forward resting your elbows on a waist-high table, or your hands on a bench (as in photograph). Have your partner sit on your lower back. (Your partner can hold a barbell plate if his/her body weight is substantially less than yours.) "Donkeys" are one of the best exercises for calf development because the weight is directly over your calves. Be sure to stretch as low as possible with your heels below the calf block. Keep your center of gravity on the balls of your feet, with your toes straight ahead. Slowly do the designated number of repetitions, stretching as low as possible, rising on your toes as high as possible and holding for one second in this top position. You will feel your calf muscles pumping and expanding. Exhale as you rise up, inhale on the way down.

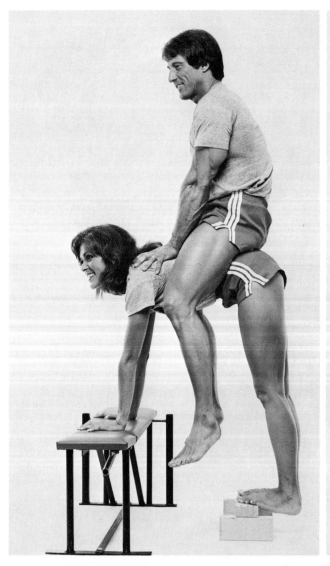
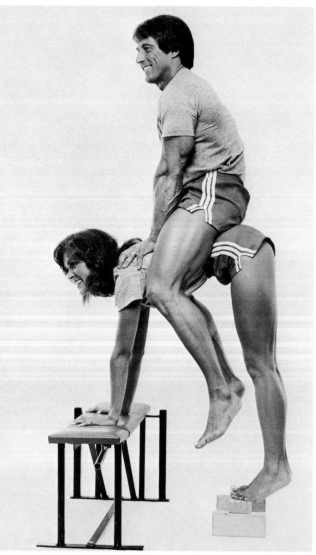

ONE-LEG CALF STRETCH

First level: 1 set, 10 sec
Middle level: 2 sets, 15 sec
Top level: 3 sets, 20 sec

Stand with one foot on a calf block with the ball of the foot touching the edge of the block. Raise high on your toes and lower as deeply as you can. Hold the stretch at the deepest point. This further stretches the lower part of the calf muscle and gives an even greater pump to this area. You will also feel the effect of this stretch in the frontal calf (tibialis). Be sure to stretch and hold as low as you can get your heel to go. Relax into the stretch, never force it.

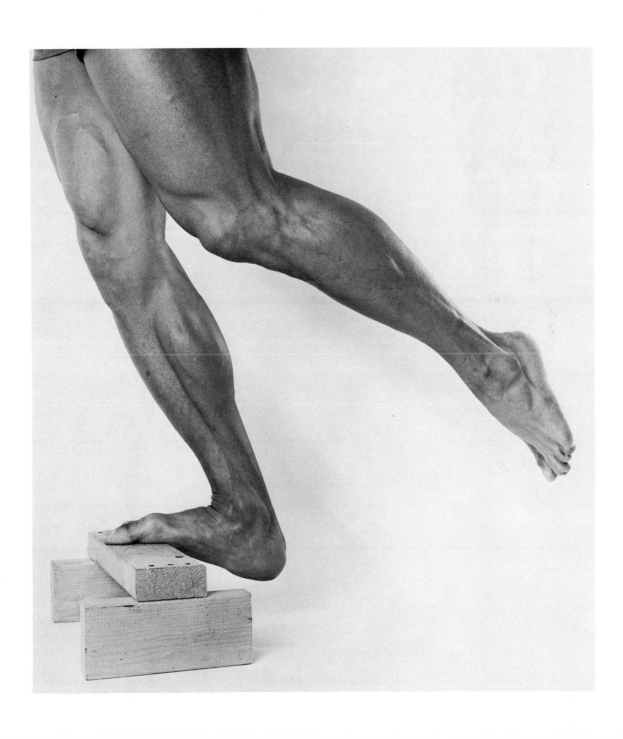

FREE-STANDING CALF RAISE

First level: 1 set, 20 reps
Middle level: 2 sets, 15 reps
Top level: 3 sets, 25 reps

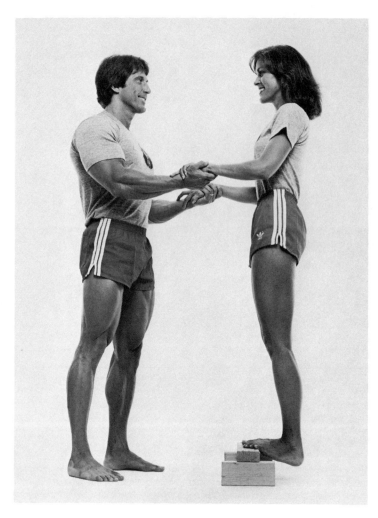

Stand on a calf block with the balls of your feet resting on the back of the block. Slowly raise up on your toes as high as you can go, pause momentarily, and then lower to the deepest possible point. Keep your balance on the balls of your feet, with your toes facing straight ahead, working all parts of your calf muscles. If you tend to slip off the block after a few reps, then simply reposition your feet. You should feel a pumping, expanding sensation in both calves after doing the repetitions.

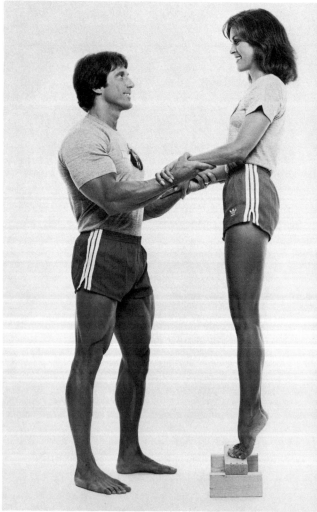

TWO-LEG CALF STRETCH

First level: 1 set, 10 sec
Middle level: 2 sets, 15 sec
Top level: 3 sets, 20 sec

Standing on a calf block with the toes of both feet resting firmly on the block, slowly raise up on your toes and lower to a very deep stretch. Hold this for the designated time and then relax. You will feel the blood circulating in the lower calves.

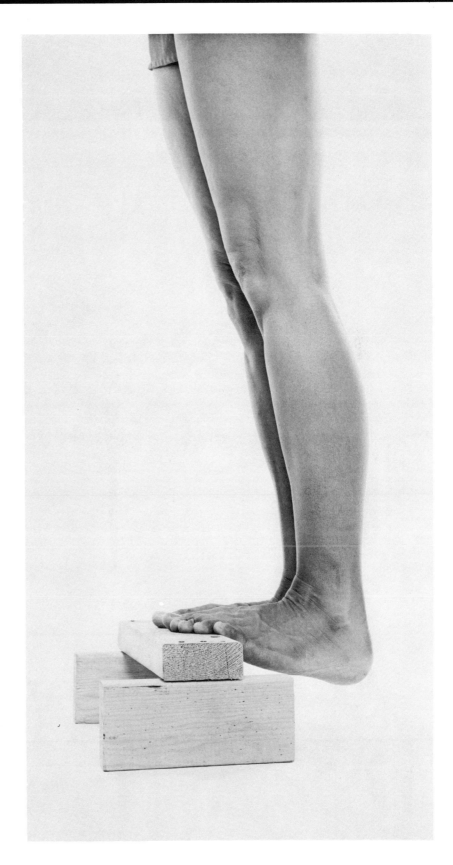

FLAT KNEE-IN

First level: 1 set, 20 reps
Middle level: 2 sets, 25 reps
Top level: 3 sets, 30 reps

Sit on the end of a flat bench so that only half of your buttocks are on the bench. Lie back and grab the legs of the bench, above your head or grasp the bench under your hips. (Grasping under the hips is slightly easier.) Bring your knees in to your chest. Exhale as you push your feet out, slightly below the level of the bench, and inhale as you bring your knees back in toward your chest. You will feel this exercise in the lower portion of your abdomen (lower rectus abdominals). Be sure to tense the abdominal muscles as the knees are pulled in to your chest.

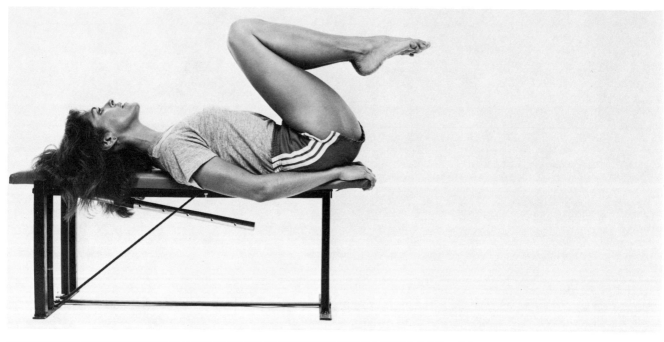

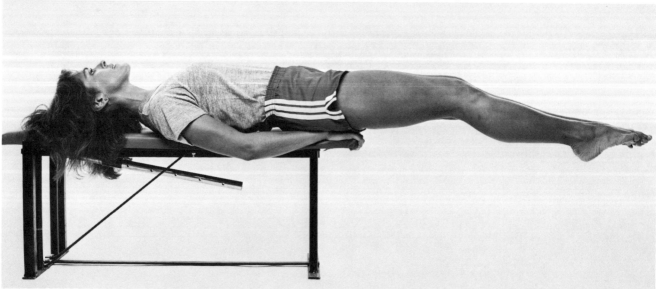

BENT-LEG PARTIAL SIT-UP

First level: 1 set, 20 reps
Middle level: 2 sets, 25 reps
Top level: 3 sets, 30 reps

Sit on the floor with your knees bent and your feet flat on the floor. Cross your arms over your chest and lie back, slowly inhaling. Exhale as you raise your buttocks off the floor and lift your back to a partial sitting position. Keep your back curved throughout the exercise. This trims and strengthens the upper abdominals. Tense the abdominals and feel the strengthening as you do each rep.

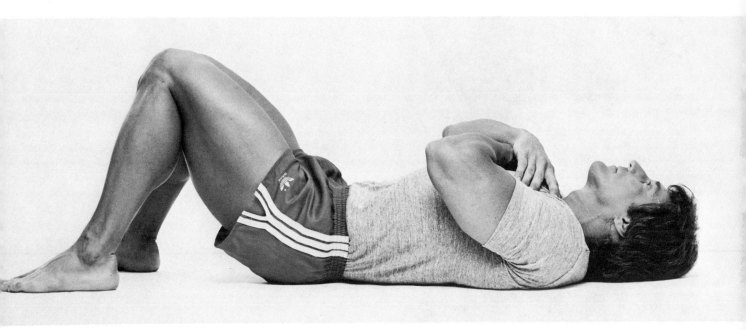

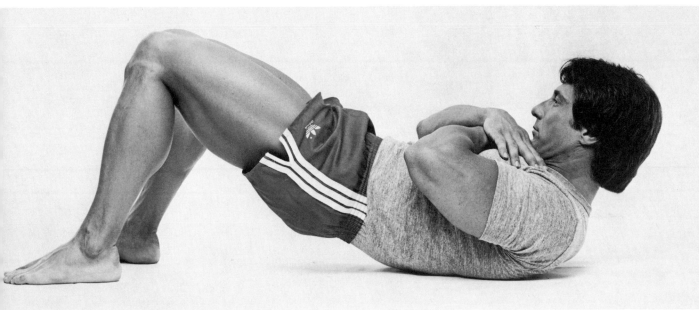

SEATED TWIST

First level: 1 set, 20 reps
Middle level: 2 sets, 25 reps
Top level: 3 sets, 30 reps

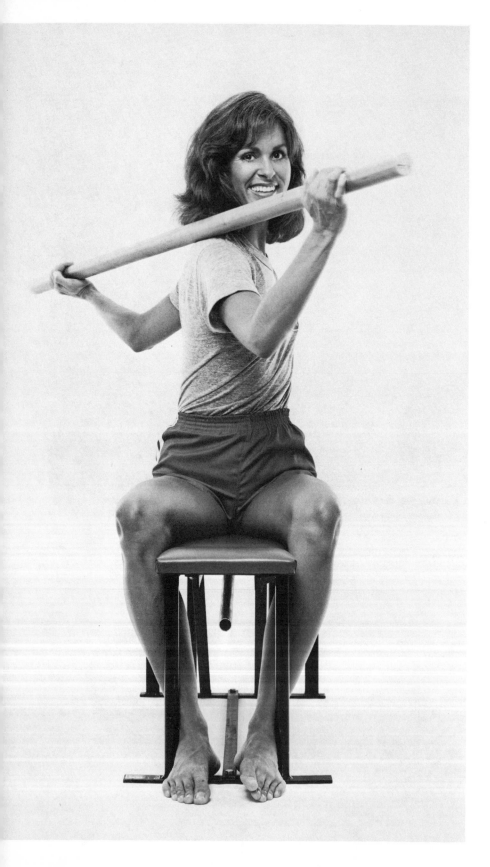

Straddle a bench and sit down. Hold a light wooden pole (like a broomstick minus the broom) across your shoulders. Keep your hips stationary and your head facing forward as you begin twisting your upper body slowly. Increase the pace to a moderate speed. This exercise is excellent for trimming the sides of your waist (intercostals and obliques) and the lower back and upper hips. You will improve twisting flexibility as you feel this movement stretching and trimming your sides.

DAILY BASIC PROGRAM
Weeks 1 to 4

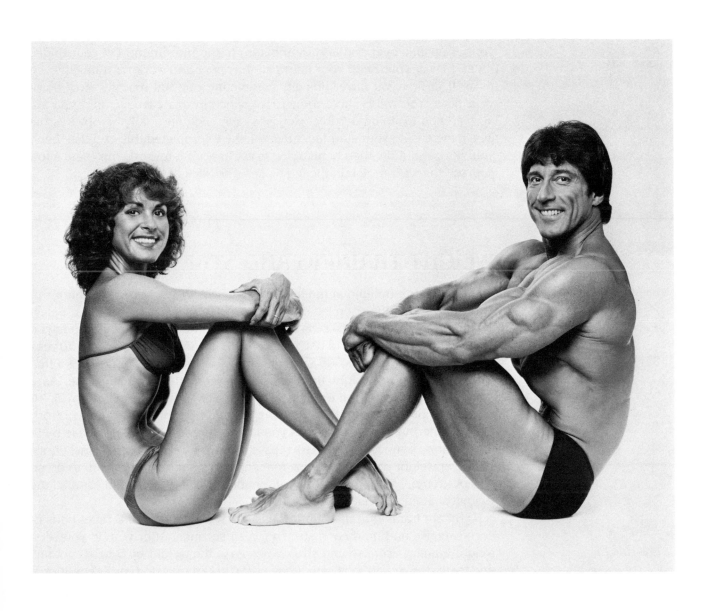

Week One
Day 1

AEROBIC EXERCISE—QUICK PACED STEP-UPS

Using a step or a well-braced bench about 10 to 15 inches high, take one full step up and one full step down. Begin slowly and increase the pace. Use a clock that is easily read while you are moving, and watch the minute hand. A kitchen timer will also work very nicely. Set the timer for 1 minute and begin your Step-ups. Proceed until the timer rings. As you do the exercise don't let your arms take over and add momentum to the movement. Let your thighs lift and lower you. Keep your knees slightly bent and work for a quick, even pace. If at first you have difficulty completing one full minute, slow down your pace. You will be able to increase speed in this exercise after you are accustomed to doing aerobic exercises daily. Regular, daily aerobics is the key to increasing your stamina. After you have completed this exercise, bend your knees slightly, then bend at the waist, reaching toward your toes. Allow yourself to feel a stretch in the leg biceps (the back of the upper legs).

WEIGHT TRAINING AND STRETCHING

Today if you are training at the first level you will do 1 set of 10 repetitions of each weight-training exercise and hold each stretch for 10 seconds. Select weights that you can do 10 reps with easily—but not too easily. It's up to you to learn what poundages to use in each exercise. If you can do 15 to 20 reps with the weight you pick, do so, but be sure to make a note of this so that you can use more weight the next time you do the same exercise. As a general rule, if any of the weights you select are too light, increase by 5, 10 or more pounds so that the repetitions can be performed with some effort. On the other hand, if the weights you choose are too heavy, decrease by 5, 10 or more pounds so that 10 reps can be performed with some effort. Whatever weight you select to use for each set, it should permit you to do no less or no more than the number of repetitions listed. This applies to all the weight-training exercises.

If you are training at the middle level you will do 2 sets of 8 repetitions of each exercise and hold each stretch for 15 seconds. After you do your first weight-training exercise and stretch, increase the weight by 5 to 10 pounds and try to do 8 repetitions with it again. If you can only do 6 or 7 repetitions,

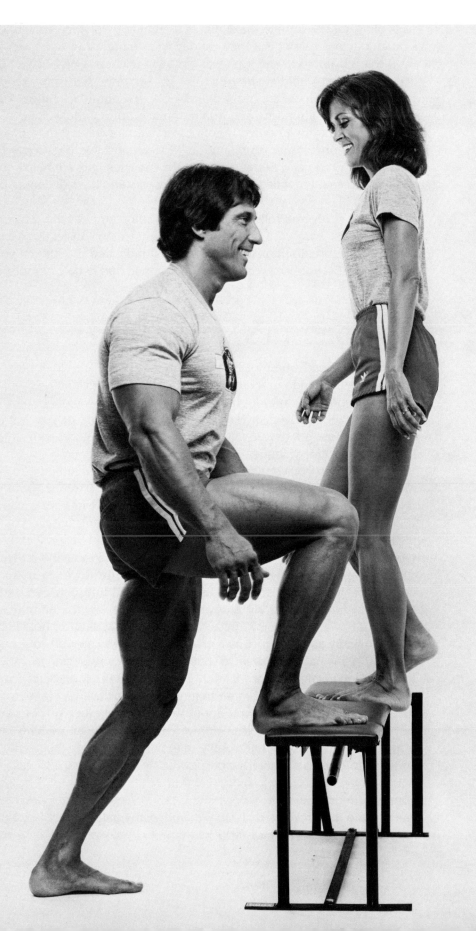

this is okay, just be sure to make a note so that you don't increase the weight as much on your second set the next day you do the exercise.

If you are training at the top level, you will do 3 sets of 12 repetitions of each exercise and hold each stretch for 20 seconds. If 12 reps on the first set was too easy, increase the weight by 5 to 10 pounds on the second set and the same for your third set. Again, make a note of the weights and reps that you use, but don't be overly concerned with increasing the weight every set; instead, concentrate on resting as little as possible between sets. This will enable you to get a better pump to the muscles and will help your body burn the excess fat that lies between the muscles and the skin (subcutaneous fat).

Be sure to study and follow the exercise photos and descriptions carefully so that you will always be aware of the correct way of doing the exercise or stretch. Where breathing instructions are not indicated, breathe in your normal manner. Do not hold your breath, but inhale and exhale smoothly.

BASIC DIET TIPS

Don't be frightened when we mention the word *diet*. We won't be speaking about a drastic change or a regimen of limited and special foods; but we will stress the importance of adopting a lifelong, healthy way of eating. There is no need to feel deprived or hungry all the time. Some of you will be very surprised at how good you will begin feeling and looking with only a few alterations to your present eating habits.

Before you can correct any habits, we feel it is of great value to become aware of how you eat now. It seems that no matter who we are, or how good we feel our eating habits are, we tend to have periods when we take a turn in the wrong direction. By becoming aware of your eating habits, you will be able to catch these tendencies more quickly before you become comfortable in an improper pattern. Get yourself a loose-leaf notebook and a pencil, and without changing your normal eating habits, write down everything that passes your lips—that means "licks" and "tastes" and between-meal "nibbles." Everything counts! Write down the time you eat, the amount, what it was, and if it was a meal or a snack. For the next five days do not change the way you usually eat. This means you will have to carry around your notebook or at least a few pages from it, so that if and when you decide to eat you can record it. Don't wait to record it later. Don't record the food before you eat it either. Often your eyes are bigger than your stomach. If you think this is too much trouble, then maybe you should reassess whether or not you really want to be aware of yourself and have the possibility of making improvements. Decide it is worth that trouble to look terrific and to feel terrific. If you can learn to exercise regularly and rigorously you can learn to eat well and healthily.

During the first week write down the foods you eat each day and read back what you ate the previous day. Do you notice any patterns, either in the time you eat or the basic type of food you eat? Do you eat meals? As you read your food record each day, think of all the reasons that this pattern of diet that you are beginning to see emerge is either working for or against you.

Reading over your food record as well as writing the foods down allows you to see clearly some of the imbalances in your diet. Most of us rely too heavily on one food group. For the majority of us, it is refined carbohydrates. These foods are easily obtainable and require little preparation. We overload on candy, sweets, cookies and fried chips. An hour or so after eating the quick-energy foods, we feel a letdown, but tend not to associate it with the sweet foods since they were eaten an hour ago. This letdown, or blood sugar drop, is caused by the sharp increase of sugar in the blood. It can be responsible for personality changes, fluctuating moods and physical weakness.

Near the third and fourth day of this week you will probably wish you could change some of the eating habits and patterns you're seeing in your diet. They may be major or they may be very minor changes, yet these patterns occur so often and add up so quickly that they slow down your progress and very often keep you from reaching your goal.

On the fifth, sixth and seventh days of this program ask yourself: "How do I feel I could effectively change my diet in minor ways that will make a noticeable difference and at the same time not cause me to feel as though I've given up everything?" In your food record write down the answers.

Day 2

AEROBIC EXERCISE

Today repeat the Quick Paced Step-ups but do them for an additional 15 seconds, for a total of 1 minute and 15 seconds. You know you can easily do 15 more seconds today. After finishing, reach up and stretch your body.

WEIGHT TRAINING AND STRETCHING

On Day 1 you exercised the muscles of the upper body: chest, shoulders, triceps, back, biceps and forearms. Today you will exercise the muscles of the lower body: thighs, calves and waist. In general, calf and waist muscles need more repetitions than upper-body muscles, for good development. If you are following the first-level program you will be doing one set of from 10 to 20 repetitions, depending on the exercise. Middle level will do two sets of 8 to 25 reps, and the top level will do three sets of from 12 to 30 repetitions. The abdominal work uses higher repetitions than either thighs or calf work. This has the effect of reducing body fat around the waist without building the abdominal muscles. Because of all the walking we've done, the calves are somewhat "stubborn" muscles on most people, and have built up a resistance to exercise. This is why the calves need more repetitions than thighs. All stretches are held for the same time as those on Day 1: 10 seconds for level one; 2 sets of 15 seconds for the middle level; and 3 sets of 20 seconds for the top level. Select your weights in the same manner as you did on Day 1, again making note of which weights you used on each set and the number of repetitions. Most of these exercises for Day 2 do not require the actual use of weights; also, the program is somewhat shorter because fewer individual areas of the body are being exercised.

Day 3

AEROBIC EXERCISE

Add 15 more seconds to your time for Quick Paced Step-ups, bringing the total time to 1 minute and 30 seconds. At the finish of this endurance-building exercise, walk slowly and take deep breaths while stretching your body.

WEIGHT TRAINING AND STRETCHING

Today you will do the same exercise program you did on Day 1. Look back on the notes you took and see which weights you used for each of the exercises and how many repetitions you did. For those exercises that were easy, use a slightly heavier weight. If you had a hard time and couldn't do the designated number of repetitions with the weight that you previously chose, lighten the weight but do each of your reps in good form. Again, make a note of which weights and repetitions you use on every set of all exercises. The amount of weight is an individual matter, so don't worry if someone is using more or less weight than you. Trying to use too much weight at first may cause injury to your muscles—and you don't want that. Be in control of the weight at all times, and you will get the most out of the weight-training movements.

If you are training at the first level, you will be holding each stretch for 10 seconds; at the middle level, for 15 seconds; and at the top level, for 20 seconds for each of the 3 sets. Do these stretches immediately after your weight-training movement. Don't force too hard during the first few seconds of each stretch; instead extend the stretch gradually, second by second. Bouncing in the stretch may cause some added tension, so don't try to bounce yourself into the full stretch; allow yourself to relax into the stretch, holding it for the designated time. With practice you will soon be able to assume the full stretch position. Stretching will give you an additional pump after the weight-training exercise, improving your flexibility.

Day 4

AEROBIC EXERCISE

Add 15 more seconds to your time for Quick Paced Step-ups for a total of 1 minute and 45 seconds, keeping a steady, comfortable pace going. Be sure to walk, breathing deeply and stretching your body after you finish.

WEIGHT TRAINING AND STRETCHING

Today you will do the same program for legs and waist as you did on Day 2. Check your notes on which weight you used for the exercises involving weights, and adjust the poundages accordingly. As before, write down the weight that you use and the number of repetitions that you do for each set. Remember, you should only be able to perform the designated number of repetitions with the weights that you select—and no more—for maximum results. Encourage your partner to do the same. Your stretching times remain the same.

Day 5

AEROBIC EXERCISE

Today you will do Quick Paced Step-ups for a total of 2 minutes. Walk and stretch after you complete the 2 minutes.

WEIGHT TRAINING AND STRETCHING

Today you repeat the Day 1 program and exercise the muscles of the upper body. Before you exercise today, visualize yourself going through each of the movements and stretches. If you forget certain exercises look them up by referring to the page numbers on the charts. Remember the weights that you used for each of the exercises. Remember, too, that your workouts are progressive: You should be adding weight as you get stronger; and you should be resting less between sets. Don't get involved in lengthy conversations between sets. Concentrate on finishing your workout without wasting time.

Day 6

AEROBIC EXERCISE

Add 15 more seconds to your time for yesterday, making your total time for Quick Paced Step-ups 2 minutes and 15 seconds. By now you should be aware that this exercise is getting easier. Your endurance is increasing. Stretch and take slow, deep breaths. Walk around a bit when you are finished.

WEIGHT TRAINING AND STRETCHING

Repeat the program for your legs and waist that you did on Day 2. This is your last workout of this week. How do you feel? If you experience a little soreness in certain areas of your body, this is okay, just so that you are not sore and stiff. If you are, then lighten your weights and do 2 or 3 more repetitions on each set. Soreness of the muscles is a sign that progress is being made. If an area of your body is very sore, do not use heavy weights in any of the exercises involving that area. Overexertion could result in increased soreness. Work for a good pump and really make this a great workout today.

Day 7

AEROBIC EXERCISE, WEIGHT TRAINING AND STRETCHING

Today is your rest day from both aerobics and weight training and stretching. Resting is as much a part of your exercise and fitness routine as are the exercises themselves. Rest enables your body to nourish and repair itself. You may feel like doing some exercises today to get ahead, but don't. If you want to participate in any of the other physical activities that you usually enjoy—like walking, tennis, bowling, golfing, swimming or playing ball—then go ahead and have fun. It's a great way to relax. You've earned a rest. so take it. You never know: Day after tomorrow you may need a rest if you exercise hard today; and remember that if you have passed up your rest day, another six days will go by before this leisure time is in your program again.

MUTUAL-ASSISTANCE TECHNIQUE

Talk to your partner today about your workouts. Criticize each other and discuss what could be done to improve them. Go over your goals. Which goals do you have in common? How can you work together to reach them? If you have any really sore areas in your body, read the section on soreness and injuries found on pp. 262–266.

Week Two
Day 8

AEROBIC EXERCISE—HIGH KICKS

Today you change aerobic exercises. Quick Paced Step-ups are replaced by High Kicks, which are a little more difficult. Not only do High Kicks condition the heart and lungs, but they also firm the thighs, waistline and calves, as well as stretch and firm the buttocks muscles. Today you will do this exercise for 1 minute. If you can't do the kicks for 1 minute without stopping, then do two segments of 30 seconds each or three segments of 20 seconds each. You will need a space that is large enough for you to extend your arms and kick each leg forward. Stand with your arms straight out in front of you, at shoulder height, with your palms facing down. Raise up on your toes and kick your right leg up to touch your fingers, and then let your leg down. Now kick the left leg up and continue alternating legs at a quick pace. Try a few

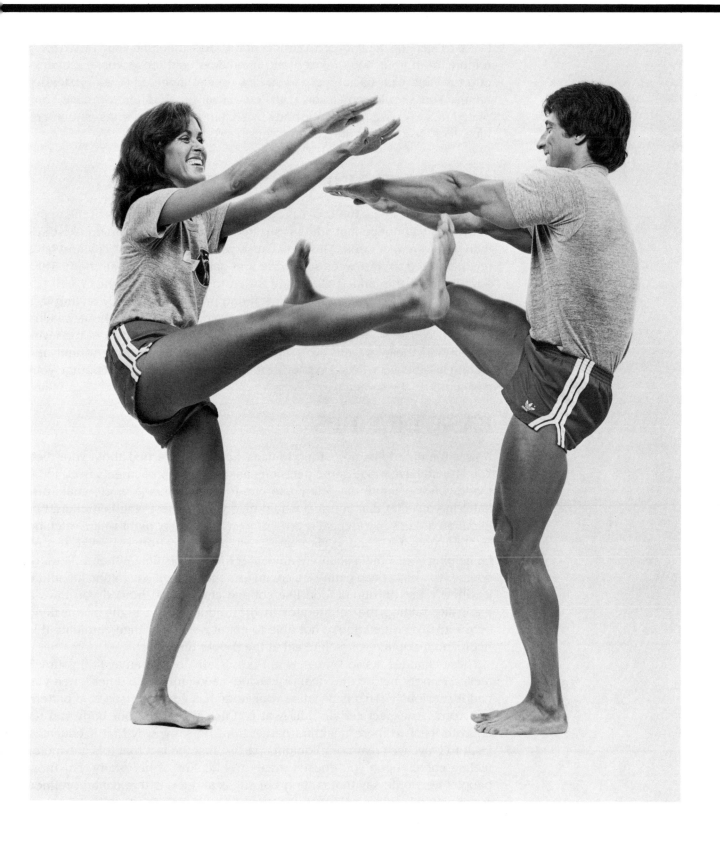

kicks to get the feeling of the movement, and then set your timer for 1 minute. With your body relaxed and shoulders held loose, make a special effort to hold your back erect as you kick up a straight leg to your extended hands. You should remain on your toes at all times. After you have completed this exercise, relax your body by shaking each part: arms, shoulders, hips, legs, feet, hands and, gently, your head.

WEIGHT TRAINING AND STRETCHING

Today you will repeat the Day-1 program and work the muscles of the upper body. You will notice that you are stronger on the weight-training exercises than you were last week. This is because you have had a rest day and have recuperated from last week's exercise and gained additional strength. Take advantage of this added vigor and strive to use more weight in all your exercises. Also, you can make your training program harder by resting less between sets. Resolve to go right through your program without wasting time between sets—whether you are training at the first, middle or top level. Remember, these are the two ways you progress: using more weight and resting less between sets. Do your best in your workouts and encourage your partner to do the same.

BASIC DIET TIPS

Now is the time to begin putting to use what you've learned about your diet. You should have made some decisions as to what improvements need to be made. On the eighth day, eliminate one food and change or eliminate one habit in your diet that you feel would give you the best results if altered or eliminated. Let's say you eat a bowl of ice cream every night while watching TV. Eliminate it. Or better, eliminate ice cream totally from your diet. It can't be helping you. Don't substitute any other food at this time either, unless, of course, you have been eating ice cream as a meal. Then you might substitute it with a more nutritious food like cottage cheese and fruit. If you have a habit like raiding the refrigerator in the middle of the night or snacking before meals so that you're not able to eat at mealtime, then eliminate this habit and discipline yourself to eat at the proper times.

These changes, as you can see, are not drastic. But you may find yourself feeling hungry before the meal or craving ice cream at the times when you had it previously. This is because your body has adapted itself to a pattern and come to expect certain things at certain times. But your body can re-educate itself to more healthful patterns in the same way that it educated itself to crave ice cream or midnight snacks. Just the fact that this craving or feeling comes upon you doesn't mean it is healthy or necessary. For most people, we would say that cutting out sugar and foods that contain refined sugar would be the wisest first alteration of their diet. Read all the labels on foods. You'll be surprised how much sugar you consume in a day. Of course, don't cut out *all* sugar products on the first day; this may be too drastic a change. Instead, do it in a gradual manner: either one food or one type of food each time. Do this every few days or weekly, whichever pattern you feel most comfortable with. These gradual changes can add up to a very healthy, strong and happy person.

Caffeine—an ingredient in colas, chocolate, coffee and many teas—would be a wise choice to eliminate. Caffeine can really play havoc with your blood sugar, often with the same effects that sugar has on your personality, energy and body appearance. The oils and acid in coffee are hard on the stomach, especially if a large amount is consumed. Too much coffee can also cause nervousness and muscular tension.

When you have made your choices this week of the changes that you will make in your diet, write them down in your records. Reread them every day. Don't allow yourself to "forget."

Day 9

AEROBIC EXERCISE

Add 15 seconds to your time for High Kicks for a total of 1 minute, 15 seconds. Begin slowly and gradually quicken the pace, striving for a straight, high kick. Try to do the full 1 minute and 15 seconds without stopping.

WEIGHT TRAINING AND STRETCHING

Repeat the Day-2 program for waistline and legs. Since you haven't exercised this area since Day 6, you should feel stronger because these areas have had time to rest and recuperate. Take advantage of this added strength and use a little more weight on all your exercises. Strive to move more quickly through your workout by resting less between sets. Do not, however, cut down on the rest times at the expense of doing each exercise correctly. Don't push yourself into the next set if you are still breathing hard. To do so would just cause sloppy form on the next exercise. Time yourself to see how long it takes to complete your workout and make a note of it. Each workout should be a little more efficient than the last.

Day 10

AEROBIC EXERCISE

High Kicks are among the more difficult aerobic exercises—but one of the great producers of results. Set your timer for 1 minute, 30 seconds (15 seconds more than yesterday) and strive to complete the exercise without stopping. As you loosen up, your kicks should get higher.

WEIGHT TRAINING AND STRETCHING

Repeat the same program that you did on Day 1 for the upper-body muscles. Today, train according to how you feel. If you feel stronger, use more weight.

If you feel capable of more endurance, rest less between sets and get a faster workout. If you feel less strength and/or endurance, then take an easier workout by cutting back on your poundages and by resting more. Be sure to make a note of the poundages and resting time, and the total length of your workout. By now you are certainly noticing some results from your exercise sessions. These results become more obvious as you continue with your regular program.

Day 11

AEROBIC EXERCISE

By now you should feel more flexibility in your thighs from High Kicks. Increase your time by 15 more seconds today for a total of 1 minute, 45 seconds. Start slowly and gradually, and try to make the full time without stopping.

WEIGHT TRAINING AND STRETCHING

Are you paying as much attention to doing your stretches correctly as you are to your weight-training exercises? Flexibility is just as important as developing the muscles; and by doing your stretches correctly, you will develop the muscles more quickly and efficiently.

Day 12

AEROBIC EXERCISE

Two minutes will be your total time for High Kicks today. Your kicks are getting easier and easier with each repetition and you have much more control over this exercise. Relax, walk around a little, and stretch after completing your 2 minutes.

WEIGHT TRAINING AND STRETCHING

Today you will repeat the Day-1 program and exercise the muscles of the upper body. Pay special attention to all your stretches and remember that when you do each stretch correctly you keep blood in the exercised area longer, giving a better pump and better development to the area. This is why One-Arm Lat Stretch should immediately follow Barbell Row: because it stretches and develops the lower lats even more.

Day 13

AEROBIC EXERCISE

Today you will go for 2 minutes, 15 seconds on your High Kicks. Pay special attention to the firming, flattening effect on the lower abdomen that this exercise produces. Don't forget to walk around and stretch after finishing.

WEIGHT TRAINING AND STRETCHING

This is your last weight-training and stretching workout for this week, so be sure to make it a good one! Today you will repeat the Day-2 program. Try to progress in any way you can over your last workout, either by using slightly more weight or by resting less and cutting down on the total length of your workout. Really concentrate on each and every exercise/stretch and feel each one working in the appropriate area.

Day 14

AEROBIC EXERCISE, WEIGHT TRAINING AND STRETCHING

You have just made it through the first 2 weeks of your new exercise program —halfway through the basic program. Congratulations! You have completed what many people consider the most difficult part of any new endeavor, the first 2 weeks. Look at what progress you have made and resolve to put energy and enthusiasm into the next week's program. Now enjoy your day of rest. You've earned it!

MUTUAL-ASSISTANCE TECHNIQUE

Have you been encouraging each other through your workouts? Every time your partner does a set immediately followed by a stretch, are you there watching and encouraging him/her? Be sure to do so if you haven't been. Are you feeling soreness in the muscles after each workout or on the following day? If you haven't been experiencing any soreness at all, try training harder by resting less or using slightly more weight (about 5 to 15 extra pounds). Your goal should be the ability to regulate how you feel after your workouts. By paying special attention to what you and your partner do during each workout, you will learn to stimulate the muscles as you want to. This control is something that will come more and more easily to you as you progress through your program.

Week Three
Day 15

AEROBIC EXERCISE—JUMP ROPE

Here's an old, familiar pastime that is remarkably good as an aerobic exercise. Jumping rope may take a little time to perfect, but just keep at it. You will soon be jumping without even one stop. As with all the other movements you have done, begin this at a slower pace and gradually step it up. You may use any style of jump you wish, as long as you make it over the rope! If you are unaccustomed to jumping rope, begin with the rope held in both hands and the loop at your heels. Rotate the rope at a fair speed until it comes over your head. As the rope nears your feet, leap, passing the rope beneath your feet and bouncing on your toes as you come down. Continue this, increasing the speed as you go. If, at first, you spend more time tangled in the rope than jumping over it, get rid of the rope and, using your imagination, go through the same motions you would if you were using the rope perfectly. You will still get the effects of jumping the rope—but you won't get all tangled up! When you jump, lift only enough to allow the rope or the imaginary rope under your feet. Adjust your timer to signal when 1 minute is over. Begin the exercise with your body relaxed. When you are finished, take some time to allow your heartbeat and breathing to return to normal. (If you must stop before the 1-minute time limit, continue your jumping when ready, for a total time of 1 minute.)

WEIGHT TRAINING AND STRETCHING

You are now beginning your third week of weight-training and stretching exercises. Continue on the same level where you have been for the first two weeks: first level, middle level, or top level. Remember that the way you progress within each of the levels is either by adding more weight or by decreasing the resting time between sets. In general, the smaller body parts like biceps, triceps, forearms, calves and even deltoids and abdominals require less rest between sets than the larger body parts like chest, back and thighs. Today you will begin your third week by repeating the Day-1 program. After you complete your workout today, compare your poundages with those you started with back on Day 1. You should be using more weight, and your total workout time should be significantly less. Really concentrate on working those upper-body muscles today!

BASIC DIET TIPS

After taking command of your desires and improving your present way of eating, you feel terrific! Continue to record your daily food intake and make a positive effort to further improve your eating habits over the next 14-day period. Think about eating more slowly. Those of us who are constantly

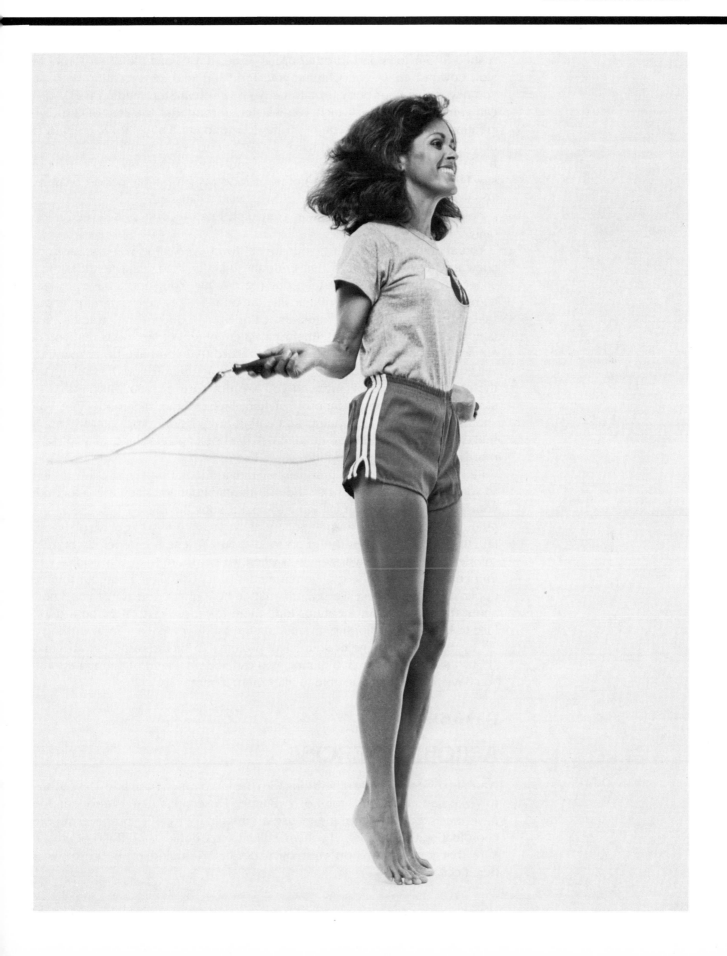

rushed in our jobs and in other areas of our day-to-day life often forget to slow down when we eat. Gulping your food can lead to overeating because you never give your body time to tell you, "I'm full! Stop feeding me!"; or it can cause indigestion, which you will feel throughout the rest of the day, creating more upsets. If you don't have time to eat a substantial meal, it is better to eat a light one and leave some time to rest and allow the food to begin to digest; or eat a smaller meal and give yourself time to eat more slowly, stretching a smaller amount of food over a longer period of time. You won't have a stuffed feeling, but you will be satisfied.

Note the gradual alterations in your diet. Keep records and reread them daily.

You should still be writing your foods down every time you eat, taste or chew anything. Even gum has enough sugar in it to make a difference, especially if you chew more than one piece a day. You should have a good, comprehensive nutrition almanac like the one the U.S. government puts out that lists all the vitamins, minerals, calories, carbohydrates, proteins, fats (saturated and unsaturated), fiber and water content of the foods that you're eating. This, accompanied by the food record that you have been keeping, will educate you about the foods that give you better nutrition. By looking up the nutritional value of anything you are not sure of, you will be able to stockpile a tremendous amount of knowledge about the foods that you should choose when shopping and eating away from home. You will soon find that only rarely will you need to use the book for reference, as you learn more about what you are eating.

Remember, continue to gradually eliminate foods that aren't contributing to your goal. Be selective. Use the nutritional almanac to see the value that your meals hold. You may want to make substitutions. Try to keep the amounts in each food group about equal. If you are trying to get rid of excess fat cut down in foods in the grain food group. These are generally high in calories and in carbohydrates; and when we eat more than our bodies can immediately use for energy, the remainder is deposited as fat on our thighs, upper arms and waist. Today, no matter how much you think you know about the foods you are eating, look them up anyway. It might be a good idea to keep a record of the groups that the foods you eat are in by putting a "P" by those that are major sources of protein, "C" by the carbohydrates and "F" by fats. In this way, at a glance, you can see what kind of eating patterns you have adopted and be able to alter them if necessary.

Day 16

AEROBIC EXERCISE

Warm up by doing a few repetitions with the jump rope. Then add 15 seconds to yesterday's time for a total of 1 minute, 15 seconds. Use the rope if you have mastered the technique or use an imaginary rope if you have trouble coordinating the exercise. If you are still having trouble using the rope, make sure that you practice on your own, because jumping rope can be very beneficial.

WEIGHT TRAINING AND STRETCHING

Today you will repeat the Day-2 program. Refer to your notes: You should notice that you are using more weight; also, the total time of your workout is somewhat shorter. Your legs and waistline should be showing some noticeable signs of definition and shaping.

Day 17

AEROBIC EXERCISES

When you Jump Rope today, sense the effect that this exercise is having on the shoulder and arm muscles. Set your timer for 1 minute, 45 seconds, and begin.

WEIGHT TRAINING AND STRETCHING

Today you will repeat the Day-1 program for the upper body. How is your upper body shaping up? Look at yourself in a two-way mirror without clothes. Are some areas firming up faster than others? What are your weak points? By now you should know which exercises in the basic program work which areas of the body; so pick the weakest part of your upper body and do an extra set of one exercise that works this area. Continue these exercises until the end of the Basic Program, which you will complete on Day 27. Don't forget to do an extra set of the stretch that also works your weakest area.

Day 18

AEROBIC EXERCISE

One minute and 45 seconds of uninterrupted jumping rope is your aim in today's aerobic exercise. Feel the exercise in your legs, especially in your calf muscles. When finished, walk around until your breathing returns to normal.

WEIGHT TRAINING AND STRETCHING

Today you will repeat the Day-2 program for your lower body. Before you begin, do as you did yesterday and look at your legs and waistline in a two-way mirror. What is your weakest area? Pick an exercise and a stretch that works this area and do an extra set until the end of the Basic Program, Day 27.

Day 19

AEROBIC EXERCISES

Today your form in Jump Rope should be better than before. Your time is now up to 2 minutes. This exercise is helping you in all those activities for which you could use more endurance and a little extra energy. All this in only 2 minutes a day!

WEIGHT TRAINING AND STRETCHING

It's back to the Day-1 program for the upper body today. Every day you are getting better and better at doing your exercises. Today pay special attention to your and your partner's form as you are doing each set. If you aren't feeling each exercise properly, in the area intended, then do each repetition more slowly, especially as you lower the weight. If you really want to feel each repetition to the maximum and gain strength faster try this system: 2 seconds to raise the weight, 1 second to hold the weight at the top of the movement when the muscle is fully contracted, and 4 seconds to lower the weight. That's a total of 7 seconds on each repetition. Your sets will take a little longer and you may have to use less weight, but you will really feel the exercise. This system can be used for all exercises or just those in which you don't feel a pump. An especially good exercise to use this system with is the Barbell Curl (p. 38).

Day 20

AEROBIC EXERCISE

Today is your last day of Jump Rope in the Basic Program. Your time is 2 minutes and 15 seconds. Begin. Notice how easy jumping rope has become for you. Walk around and stretch after finishing.

WEIGHT TRAINING AND STRETCHING

This is your last workout of Week 3. If you compare the weights you were using when you started with those you are handling now, you will notice that there is a significant difference. Your workout time is shorter now as well. Training with fewer rests between sets has a good cardiovascular effect as well as shaping and firming your muscles. Tomorrow you have a day of rest to look forward to, so make this a great workout!

Day 21

AEROBIC EXERCISE, WEIGHT TRAINING AND STRETCHING

You've made it through your third week of the program. By now you're becoming more aware of what each exercise does for you. For the next week continue to do an extra set of whichever weight-training exercise and stretch that works your weakest areas. Try to add weight on this extra set if you are training at the first or middle levels. If you are training at the top level, keep the same weight you had on your third set but rest very little before going on to the last set. This coming week you will be better than ever at your program—stronger, with more endurance, and looking and feeling better than before.

MUTUAL-ASSISTANCE TECHNIQUE

You can make even faster progress and cut down on unwanted body fat if you improve your diet. Because our bodies are nourished and maintained by the foods we eat, what we eat eventually becomes a part of us. Now is a good time to start thinking about how you and your partner can help each other to continue cleaning up your diets. Discuss this with your partner.

Week Four
Day 22

AEROBIC EXERCISE—TRACK START

Your aerobic exercise this week resembles the starting position taken by many track athletes when taking off from the starting point. To get into this position for the Track Start, first look at the photo and study it carefully. Next place your feet together and bend over at the waist, bending the knees until you are in a squatting position, with the palms of your hands to each side, and in front of your feet. Keep your left leg bent and stretch your right foot back until the knee is nearly straightened. The toes of your right foot should only be touching the floor and your left foot should be as flatly planted as possible. If your Achilles tendon is stiff this exercise may be a little more of a challenge for you, and we suggest that you stretch your tendon out by standing up and raising your toes upward. Or for a deeper stretch, place your toes on a step and stretch down as far as is comfortable. Try this before each aerobic session this week. This stretch is like a negative calf raise. Get back into the starting position. With a slight bounce to push your body, push your left leg back and bring your right leg up to the position your left foot just held, behind your right hand. Begin the movement slowly and continue alternating legs, forward and back. After a few repetitions, set your timer for 1 minute. Take a deep breath and begin the exercise. Keep a fairly fast pace throughout the minute. One important detail to remember is to place your feet in about the same place each time. Get the maximum stretch. After you are finished, shake your body out, breathe and walk slowly until you are relaxed and your heart rate has returned to near normal.

WEIGHT TRAINING AND STRETCHING

Today you should feel well rested and strong after your day of rest. If you don't you may be overtraining or overdoing your workouts. If you feel tired instead of invigorated, then drop back to the Middle Level if you are at the Top Level, or to the First Level is you are training at the Middle Level, and rest more between sets if you are at the First Level. Do this for one week only and then resume your former level. Today pay special attention to the way you feel, and if you are strong, take advantage of your condition by using a little more weight.

BASIC DIET TIPS

You should still be keeping track of what you eat as well as eliminating those foods that will not help you reach your goal. By now, we hope you have eliminated all refined sugars, and sugar in general unless they are from fresh fruits and dairy products—and refined flours. Instead of refined grain, you should use whole grains in moderation. Refined oils, such as margarine

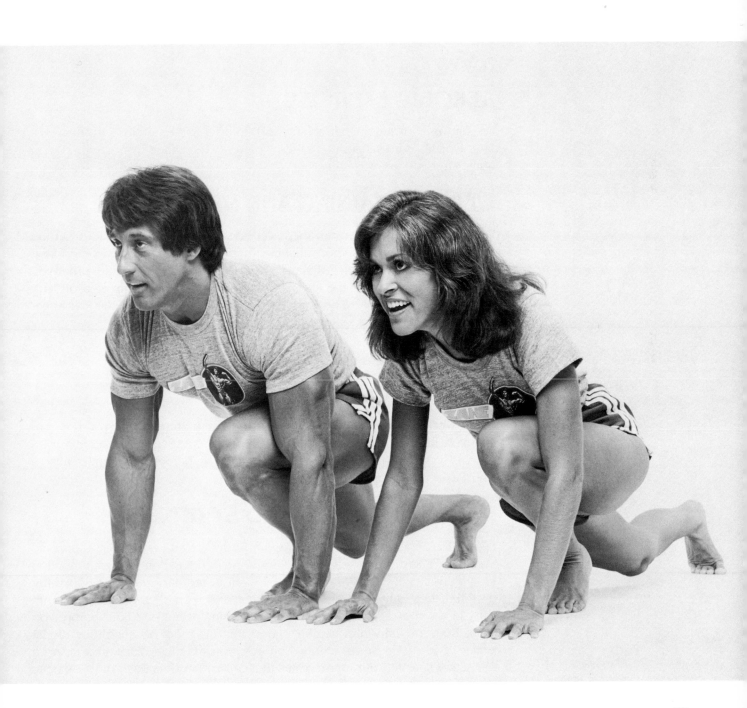

and shortening should be eliminated; use small amounts of butter instead and clarified butter for cooking. You can find out how to make clarified butter in just about any cookbook. You will notice that your food is tastier when it isn't hidden under a lot of "processes." Your shopping will be easier too. You will be spending less time in the market going up and down the endless aisles of overly processed, canned, frozen and boxed foods and will only have to go to the fresh food sections. Remember that processed, canned, frozen and boxed foods have lost a lot of nutrients by the time they get to you. Fresh foods take less time to prepare; and if you buy foods that are in season, you will also end up saving money.

Day 23

AEROBIC EXERCISE

Loosen up your legs by stretching and doing a few repetitions of the Track Start slowly. Then set your timer for 1 minute, 15 seconds, and begin. Warm down after you are done.

WEIGHT TRAINING AND STRETCHING

Repeat the Day-2 program for the lower body. Can you feel your legs getting stronger and firmer? Is your waistline shaping up the way you would like it to? If not, add another set of waist exercises that reaches the area that you want to improve. Since the lower part of the waist is sometimes a difficult area to improve, it might be a good idea to do an extra set of the Flat Knee-in (p. 52) to hasten the shape-up process.

Day 24

AEROBIC EXERCISE

Today work on perfecting your form in the Track Start so that you feel that you have sufficiently worked your entire system after completing the 1 minute, 30 second time period. Be sure to loosen up before you exercise and to warm down afterward.

WEIGHT TRAINING AND STRETCHING

Repeat the Day-1 program for the upper body. Are you exercising at approximately the same time each day? Setting a regular time for your training session makes it easier to get into the habit of regular exercise. Choose the time that best suits you and your partner and then stick to it. If you train early in the morning, be sure to eat something about one hour before you train. Eggs or dairy products are good for this meal because they digest easily. If you train on an empty stomach, you may feel dizzy after doing a few sets, especially during exercises that call for bending over, or if you have to lie down and get up. Eating prior to a workout helps keep your blood sugar up and gives you a better pump.

Day 25

AEROBIC EXERCISE

This is an excellent movement which will give you the endurance, speed and agility needed for every sport. In your weight training, Track Start can be used as a stretching movement along with your leg workouts. Today you are doing them for your circulatory system and lungs. You'll want the pace to be quick and regular. It is easier and easier to do, the more practice you get. Set your timer for 1 minute, 45 seconds, and begin.

WEIGHT TRAINING AND STRETCHING

Today you will be exercising your legs and waist with the Day-2 program. By now you should be familiar with all the exercises in both upper- and lower-body programs. It is a good idea to have all the exercises that you are going to do written down in a notebook so that you can go right through your workout writing down the weights, sets and reps. Written records are valuable because you can refer back to previous workouts and can use them to help you get into shape in the future.

Day 26

AEROBIC EXERCISE

Today you will do the Track Start for 2 minutes. Visualize a brand new "motor" running in your body that makes you feel lighter and more energetic than ever before. After you have completed the exercise, walk around and stretch to warm down.

WEIGHT TRAINING AND STRETCHING

Repeat your Day-1 program. You have probably noticed that your strength and energy vary from day to day. Not getting enough sleep, improper nutrition, excessive mental preoccupation, stress can affect the way you feel and train. If you have any negative thoughts, try to put them away during your workout and you will find that your exercises will go better and that your attitude will become more positive and stay with you for the rest of the day. If you notice your partner having a "low" day, give him/her moral support and encourage him/her to have a better workout.

Day 27

AEROBIC EXERCISE

Push your time for Track Start up to 2 minutes, 15 seconds. This is your last aerobic workout of this week, so make it count by concentrating on getting a full extension as you step forward with each leg.

WEIGHT TRAINING AND STRETCHING

Today is your last day to work out on the Basic Program. Next week you move up to the Intermediate Program, so really give this lower-body workout (repeating Day-2 program) everything you've got! As you do your exercises today, notice how much stronger your legs have become.

Day 28

AEROBIC EXERCISE, WEIGHT TRAINING AND STRETCHING

Get out and do something different today. A change of scenery would be excellent, so think about a short trip or some recreational exercise.

You have completed your first month's program and have improved in health, strength, stamina and appearance in ways you don't even realize. You have started on a trend of improvement which will become more and more apparent to you and others as you continue to progress through the Intermediate Program and the Advanced Program that lie ahead. Relax and have a wonderful time today.

MUTUAL-ASSISTANCE TECHNIQUE

By now you should be keeping a workout journal or diary. You can combine it with your food record or keep it separately. During each workout, between sets or immediately afterward, write down what you did in your workout. Copy the schedule you will be doing each day and write down weights, sets and reps.

Next to each exercise, every time you do more than you've done previously —if you've used more weight or done more reps or sets—put a star by the exercise. Score at least one star per workout. At the end of this week, and every week following, review your workouts and plan the weights and reps that you'll use next week. Look over what you've done and decide how you can improve your workout.

BASIC PROGRAM	First Level			Middle Level			Top Level		
Day-1 Exercises	Weight Used	Sets	Reps	Weight Used	Sets	Reps	Weight Used	Sets	Reps
Push-ups (warm-up)									
Bench Press									
Doorway Stretch									
Dumbbell Pullover									
Overhead Stretch									
Press Behind Neck									
One-Arm Shoulder Stretch									
Barbell Row									
One-Arm Lat Stretch									
Close-Grip Bench Press									
Arms-Backward Stretch									
Barbell Curl									
Arms-Backward Stretch with Pronation									
Reverse Curl									
Fist Curl, Wrist Down									

BASIC PROGRAM	First Level			Middle Level			Top Level		
Day-2 Exercises	Weight Used	Sets	Reps	Weight Used	Sets	Reps	Weight Used	Sets	Reps
One-Leg Top Extension (warm-up)									
Half Squat									
Lunge with Back Foot on Bench									
Lunge on Step									
Forward Stretch									
Donkey Calf Raise									
One-Leg Calf Stretch									
Free-Standing Calf Raise									
Two-Leg Calf Stretch									
Flat Knee-in									
Bent-Leg Partial Sit-up									
Seated Twist									

This chart (also found at the end of the Intermediate and Advanced sections) can be used to keep track of your progress.

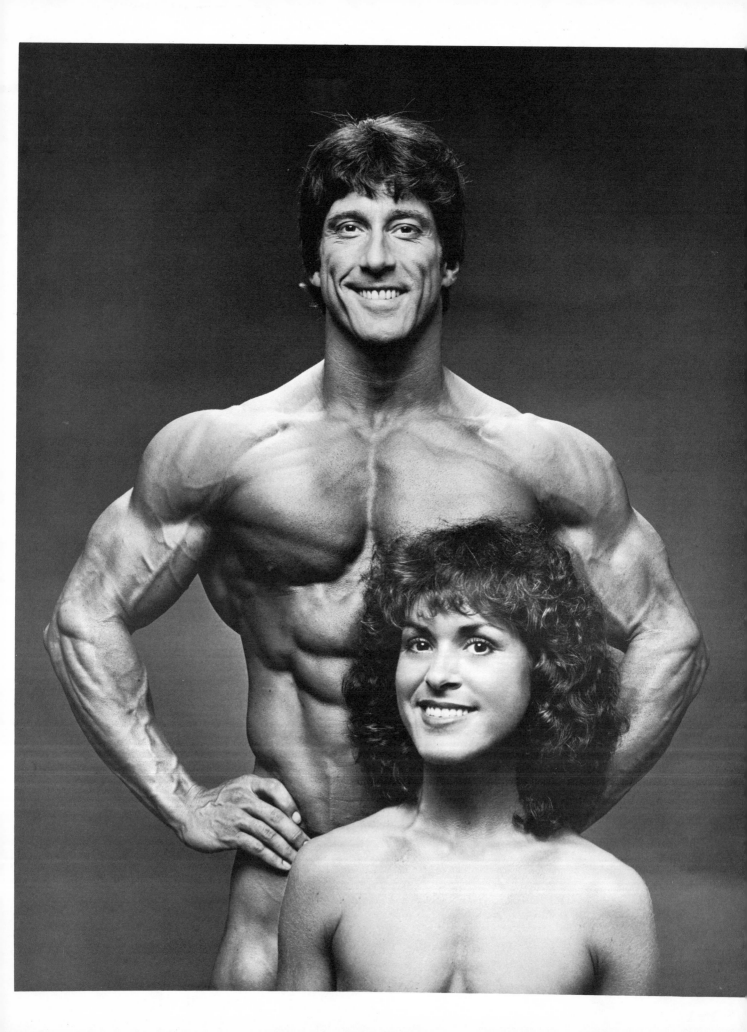

INTERMEDIATE
PROGRAM

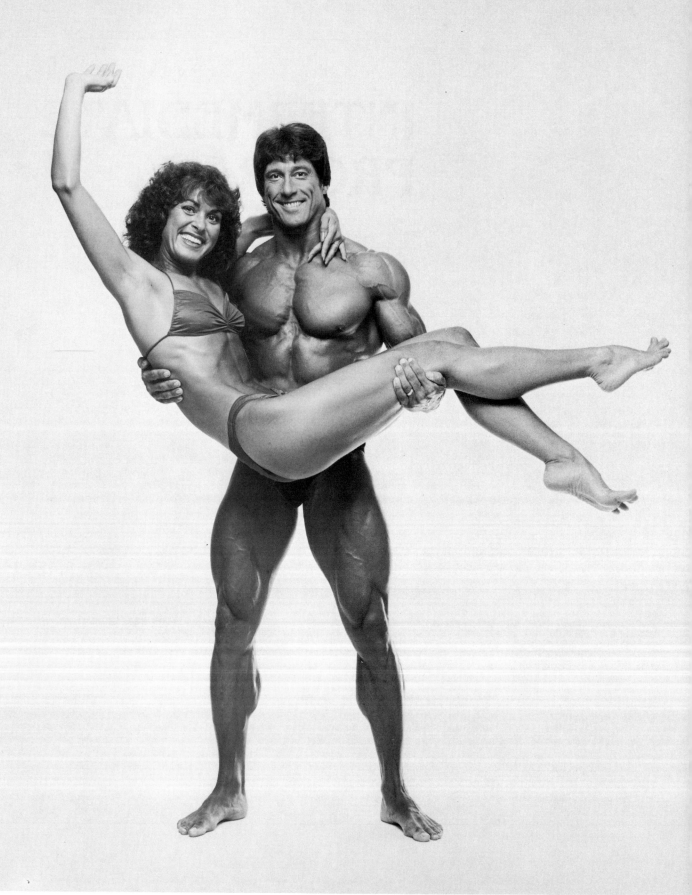

Introduction

Now you are ready for the Intermediate Program. Whether you are following the program at the first, middle or top level, you are undoubtedly becoming stronger. You should have on hand enough weight so that the dumbbells go up to 55 pounds each and a barbell up to 200 pounds total weight. Go by the poundages you used in the Basic Program in order to get a good idea of how much weight you will need now. You will also need an overhead bar. This is the only additional equipment required for the Intermediate Program.

The aerobic exercises you will be doing the next 4 weeks become progressively more difficult. The time allotted to finish the exercise will begin at 2 minutes, with 15-second increases each day. Even if you do a lot of jogging or running, go through the daily aerobic-type exercises that we give as well. They are designed to work other parts of the body, along with conditioning your heart, lungs and circulatory system.

The Intermediate weight-training program incorporates more exercises into each daily workout. The Basic Program had 7 weight exercises and 8 stretches one day and 8 exercises and 4 stretches the following day, and then repeated each session twice more during the week. Now you will be doing 9 weight-training exercises and 7 stretches one day, 10 exercises and 7 stretches the next day, followed by 9 exercises and 5 stretches the following day. Each of these 3 sessions is repeated one more time during the week. In the Basic Program each body part was worked 3 times a week. In the Intermediate Program each body part, except the waist, is worked twice a week, but more work is done for each area per workout. The waist is worked 6 days a week, which will make it smaller and tighter in a shorter time.

In the Intermediate Program you will continue to do most of the weight-training exercises you did in the Basic Program; but some new ones will be added to work the body from different angles, giving more complete physical development. Remember to do your stretching movement immediately after each set of weight-training exercises. Some new stretches will be added here as well.

Your strength and endurance are increasing, so don't hesitate to use more weight as you feel stronger. Conversely, if the weights you choose feel too heavy use less weight. As you progress through the Intermediate Program, you should be cutting down to 1½- or 2-minute rest periods between sets.

One of the many advantages of couples training is that it becomes easier to set and maintain a proper pace. *Pace* is the length of time it takes to complete a cycle of weight-training exercises, stretching and rest—in that order. Your pace should stay constant throughout the workout. This is because one person is resting while the other is doing a set of weight-training exercises and the stretching movement. Encourage each other to move through the training session, and keep your conversation to a minimum—speaking only words of encouragement to your partner.

Leaner doesn't necessarily mean skinnier. (By leaner we mean the amount of fat surrounding the muscle.) Losing fat does not also mean losing muscle. When you lose a good amount of this excess fat in the next 4 weeks you may be surprised. You may not have as much muscle as you thought you did.

Body awareness means seeing and knowing exactly what your body looks like at all times. We will give you some exercises that will help you see yourself in a clearer light. You will be doing exercises in your mind and on paper which will involve visual, auditory and kinesthetic modes of experience. Give these methods a chance. We feel that they are an integral part of the entire program. You will begin noticing an acceleration in your progress. Your body will become noticeably different each week. A Mutual-Assistance Technique along with Diet and Nutritional Tips will continue to be given weekly.

The care you're now taking of your body will continue to pay off for the rest of your life. Do your program and reach for your goal with this in mind.

Here is the first part of your new Intermediate Program. Over the course of the next month this program is to be followed on Days 29, 32, 36, 39, 43, 46, 50 and 53. These exercises will work your back, biceps, forearms and abdominal muscles.

EXERCISE	Page	First Level	Middle Level	Top Level
Dumbbell Shrug	86	1 set, 10 reps	2 sets, 8 reps	3 sets, 12 reps
Downward Neck Stretch	87	10 seconds	2 sets, 15 sec	3 sets, 20 sec
Wide-Grip Chins or Letdowns	88	1 set, 10 reps	2 sets, 8 reps	3 sets, 12 reps
Sideways Swing	90	1 set, 10 reps	2 sets, 8 reps	3 sets, 12 reps
Barbell Row	91	1 set, 10 reps	2 sets, 8 reps	3 sets, 12 reps
One-Arm Lat Stretch	91	10 seconds	2 sets, 15 sec	3 sets, 20 sec
Barbell Curl	92	1 set, 10 reps	2 sets, 8 reps	3 sets, 12 reps
Arms Backward Stretch with Pronation	92	10 seconds	2 sets, 15 sec	3 sets, 20 sec
Alternate Dumbbell Curl	93	1 set, 10 reps	2 sets, 8 reps	3 sets, 12 reps
Push-ups, Fingers Back Stretch	94	10 seconds	2 sets, 15 sec	3 sets, 20 sec
Wrist Curl	95	1 set, 10 reps	2 sets, 8 reps	3 sets, 12 reps
Wall Lean (for forearms)	96	10 seconds	2 sets, 15 sec	3 sets, 20 sec
Reverse Curl	97	1 set, 10 reps	2 sets, 8 reps	3 sets, 12 reps
Fist Curl, Wrist Down	97	10 seconds	2 sets, 15 sec	3 sets, 20 sec
Incline Knee-in	98	1 set, 20 reps	2 sets, 25 reps	3 sets, 30 reps

DUMBBELL SHRUG

First level: 1 set, 10 reps
Middle level: 2 sets, 8 reps
Top level: 3 sets, 12 reps

This exercise works the trapezius muscles of the upper back. It is especially good for developing vertical height to the traps and strengthening the neck. Let the dumbbells slide up the front of your thighs, and hold the shrug 1 second before letting your shoulders slowly drop. You will really feel the blood circulation in the upper back and neck areas. Immediately after Dumbbell Shrug, do Downward Neck Stretch.

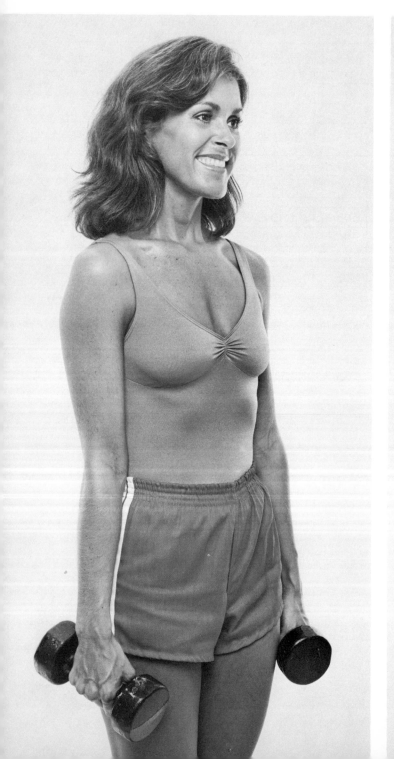
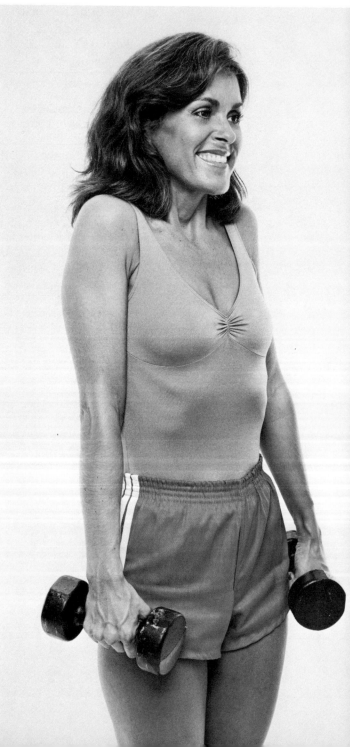

DOWNWARD NECK STRETCH

First level: 1 set, 10 sec
Middle level: 2 sets, 15 sec
Top level: 3 sets, 20 sec

Bend your head down as far as it will go and hold for a count of 10 to 20 seconds. You will really feel a stretching, muscle-relaxing sensation in the back of your neck. People hold a lot of tension in the upper back—neck area, and shrugs along with neck stretches are a good way to bring a fresh blood supply to this area and work out the tension.

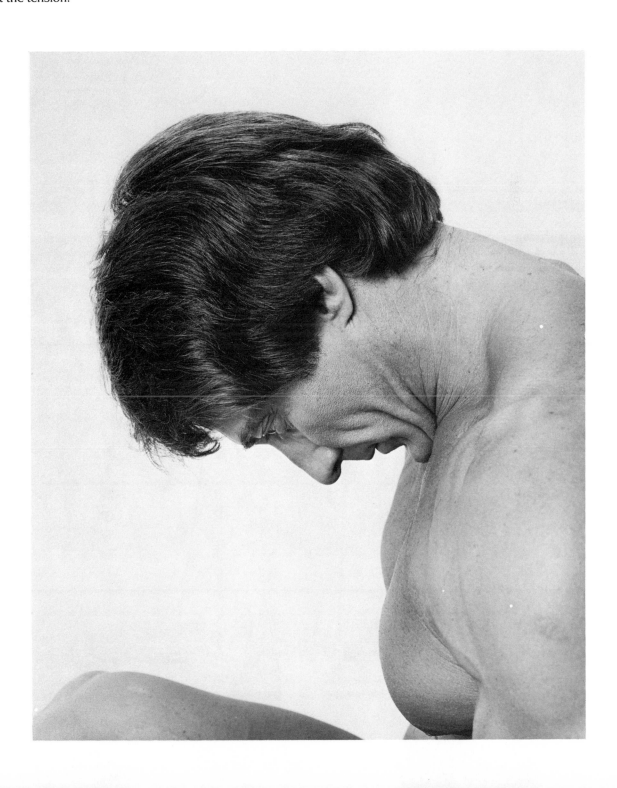

WIDE-GRIP CHINS or LETDOWNS

First level: 1 set, 10 reps
Middle level: 2 sets, 8 reps
Top level: 3 sets, 12 reps

These two exercises develop width to the upper back. Do them with a thumbless grip grasping an overhead bar with your hands 3 to 4 feet apart. For Wide-Grip Chins pull yourself up to the bar until your chin touches. Lower slowly and repeat. You should be able to do at least 8 to 10 reps. If you can only do 3 or 4 reps, try Letdowns. Have your partner boost you up until your chin touches the bar. Then on your own, hold for 1 second and take a good 4 seconds to slowly lower yourself. This will help you build up enough strength to do chins. Your shoulders and back will feel wider after doing this. As soon as you finish your last rep do Sideways Swing.

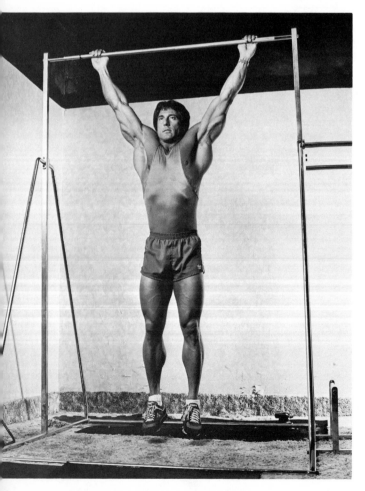
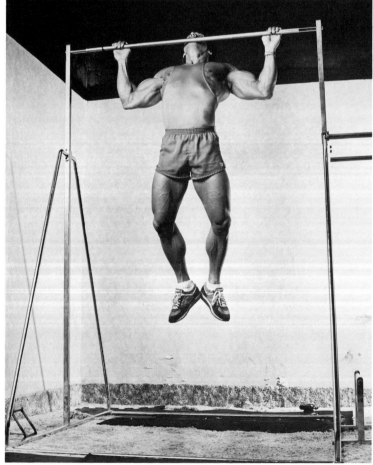

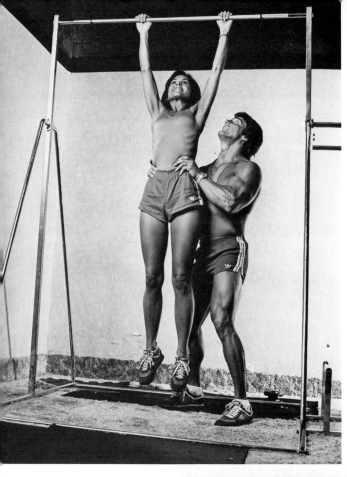

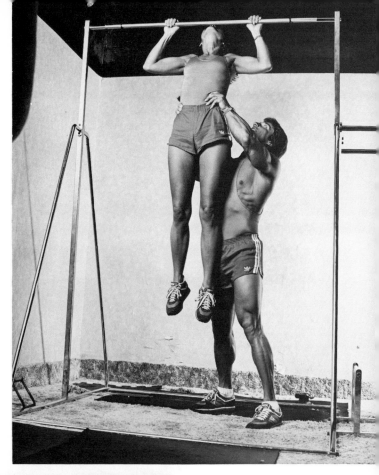

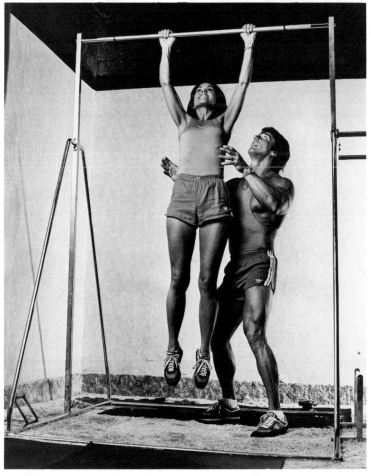

SIDEWAYS SWING

First level: 1 set, 10 reps
Middle level: 2 sets, 8 reps
Top level: 3 sets, 12 reps

With a wide grip, swing to your left and then right the designated number of times. This really stretches the lats and serratus.

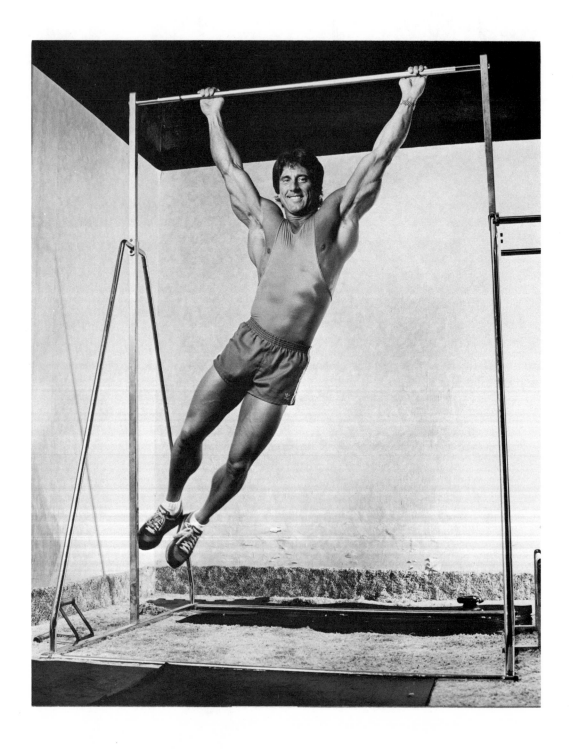

90

BARBELL ROW

First level: 1 set, 10 reps
Middle level: 2 sets, 8 reps
Top level: 3 sets, 12 reps

ONE-ARM LAT STRETCH

First level: 1 set, 10 sec
Middle level: 2 sets, 15 sec
Top level: 3 sets, 20 sec

This is an exercise/stretch sequence you followed in the Basic Program. The most important part of Barbell Row is to lower the weight slowly until it almost touches the floor and rounds your back. With the barbell in this position your lower lats are stretched to the maximum. You'll feel a terrific pump in your entire back. Doing the exercise in this way, if you do the One-Arm Lat Stretch immediately afterward, you'll feel an even deeper stimulation in this same area. Really stretch with both right and left arms.

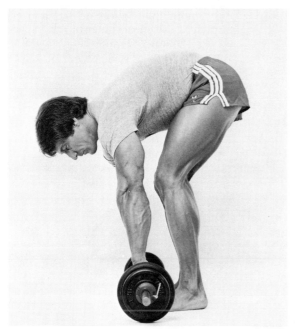
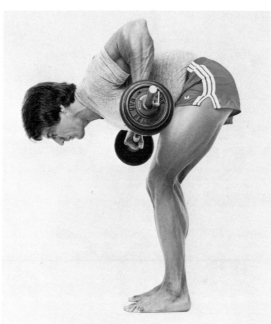
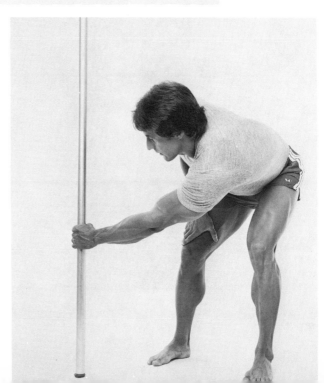

BARBELL CURL

First level: 1 set, 10 reps
Middle level: 2 sets, 8 reps
Top level: 3 sets, 12 reps

ARMS BACKWARD STRETCH with PRONATION

First level: 1 set, 10 sec
Middle level: 2 sets, 15 s
Top level: 3 sets, 20 sec

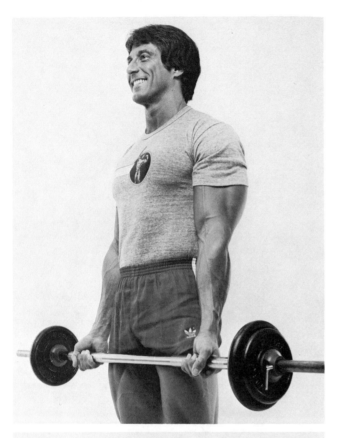

This movement is a great overall biceps developer. Do this exercise the same way you did it in your Basic Program. Make sure that your arms completely straighten out as you start each repetition. This part of the curl works the lower part of the biceps. Also, don't allow the weight to fall in at the top of the movement. Keep your wrists straight. You should tense the biceps in this position and then slowly lower the barbell until the arms are completely straight. Your forearms develop from this exercise as well. Also do Arms Backward Stretch with Pronation as before in the Basic Program. Try to pronate, or turn the wrist inward, even more than before to get a good stretch to the lower, outer biceps as well as the forearms. This stretch should always be done along with any biceps work.

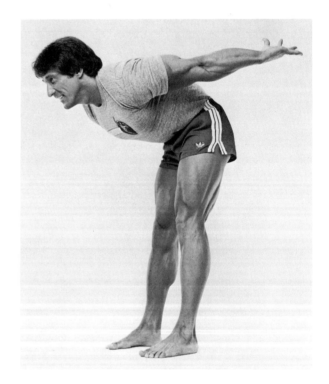

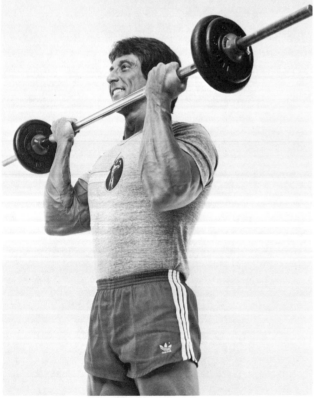

92

ALTERNATE DUMBBELL CURL

First level: 1 set, 10 reps
Middle level: 2 sets, 8 reps
Top level: 3 sets, 12 reps

Stand with a dumbbell in each hand. Keep your elbows close to each side. Inhale and raise one dumbbell up, keeping your wrist straight, and turn the dumbbell so your palms are facing up and the dumbbell is held horizontal in the finish position. Lower the dumbbell slowly, turning your wrist in as you do. Repeat this motion with the other arm and continue to alternate. As you curl the weight up, you work the outer biceps; and as you lower the weight, you work your forearms.

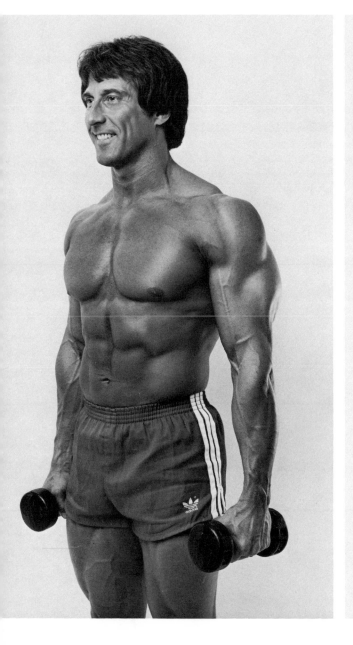
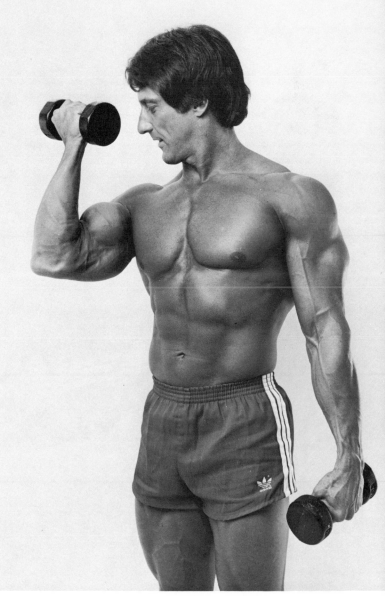

93

PUSH-UPS, FINGERS BACK STRETCH

First level: 1 set, 10 sec
Middle level: 2 sets, 15 sec
Top level: 3 sets, 20 sec

Lie on the floor as you did for Push-ups. Turn your hands so that your fingers are pointing backward toward your feet. Hold this position for the designated time, then relax. You should really feel this stretch in your forearms.

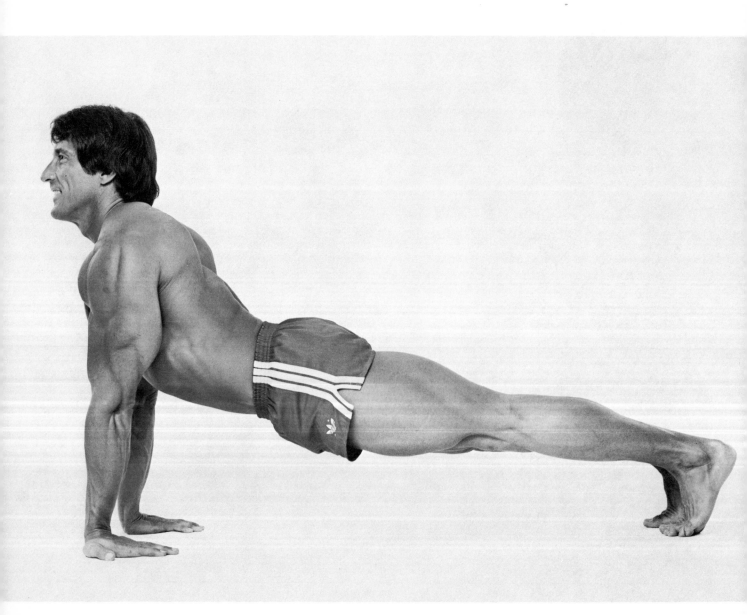

WRIST CURL

First level: 1 set, 10 reps
Middle level: 2 sets, 8 reps
Top level: 3 sets, 12 reps

Sit on the end of a bench with your wrists resting on your knees, palms facing up. Hold a barbell with a thumbless grip, and slowly curl your fists up and in. Hold this position for a second and lower your fists into the down position. Don't allow the barbell to roll down your fingers. Don't put your thumbs around the bar. You should feel Wrist Curls in the palm side of your forearms. Work for a good pump in this exercise and then go on to the following exercise.

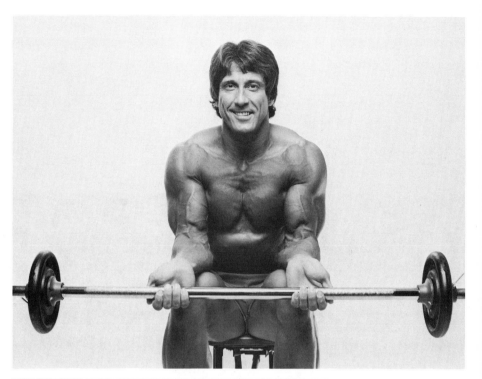

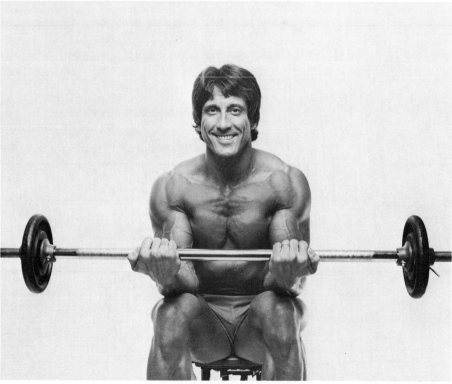

95

WALL LEAN

First level: 1 set, 10 sec
Middle level: 2 sets, 15 sec
Top level: 3 sets, 20 sec

Stand facing a wall. Allow about 1 foot of space between you and the wall for each foot of your height. Keep your feet flat and lean forward with your palms flat on the wall at chest level. Push until you feel the stretch in your calves and forearms. Pay special attention to and concentrate on the forearms stretching. If you don't feel a stretch, adjust your body nearer or farther away from the wall until you do. Hold the stretch before relaxing.

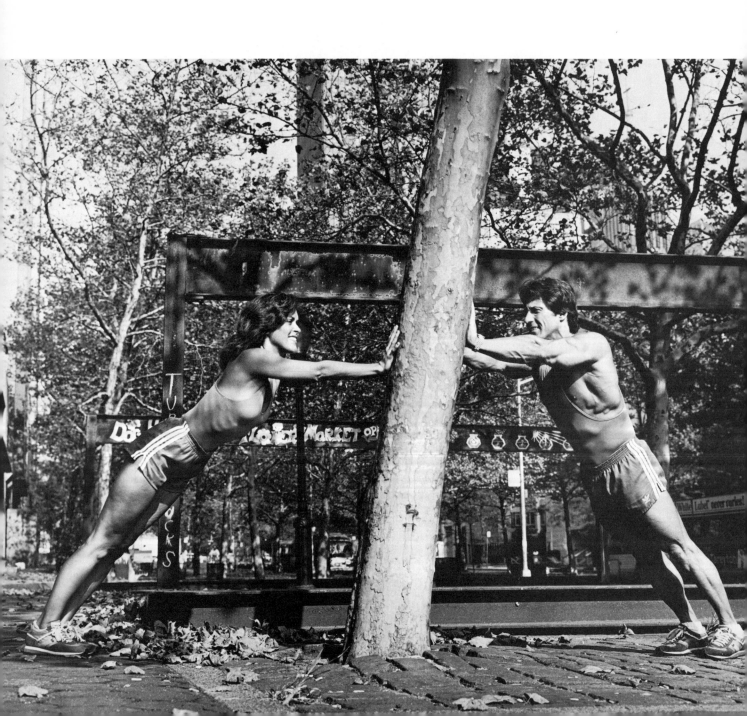

REVERSE CURL

First level: 1 set, 10 reps
Middle level: 2 sets, 8 reps
Top level: 3 sets, 12 reps

FIST CURL, WRIST DOWN

First level: 1 set, 10 sec
Middle level: 2 sets, 15 sec
Top level: 3 sets, 20 sec

In your workout today, continue to do these two exercises (which immediately follow Wall Lean) as you have been doing all along. Your grip should be much stronger. This is of immense value in sports such as baseball, tennis and golf. For an added effect, squeeze the barbell during the last few repetitions of Reverse Curl. This will further strengthen your grip and develop your forearms. Refer back in the book to these two exercises to make sure that you're doing them correctly.

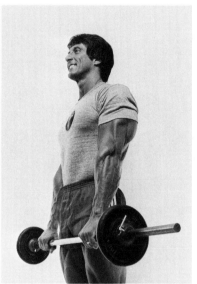 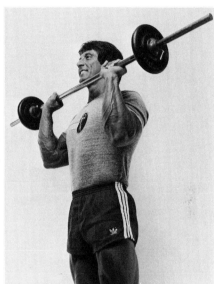

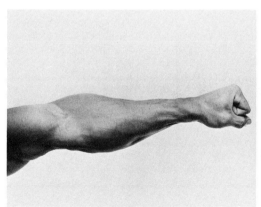 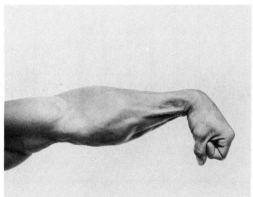

INCLINE KNEE-IN

First level: 1 set, 20 reps
Middle level: 2 sets, 25 reps
Top level: 3 sets, 30 reps

Prop a flat bench up on a calf block to form an incline. Lie on the safely secured bench and do the exercise in the same way you did Flat Knee-in (p. 52) in the Basic Program. This exercise tightens the abdominal area at the navel and below. This is where fat accumulates easily. Keep your abdominal muscles flexed as you do each repetition.

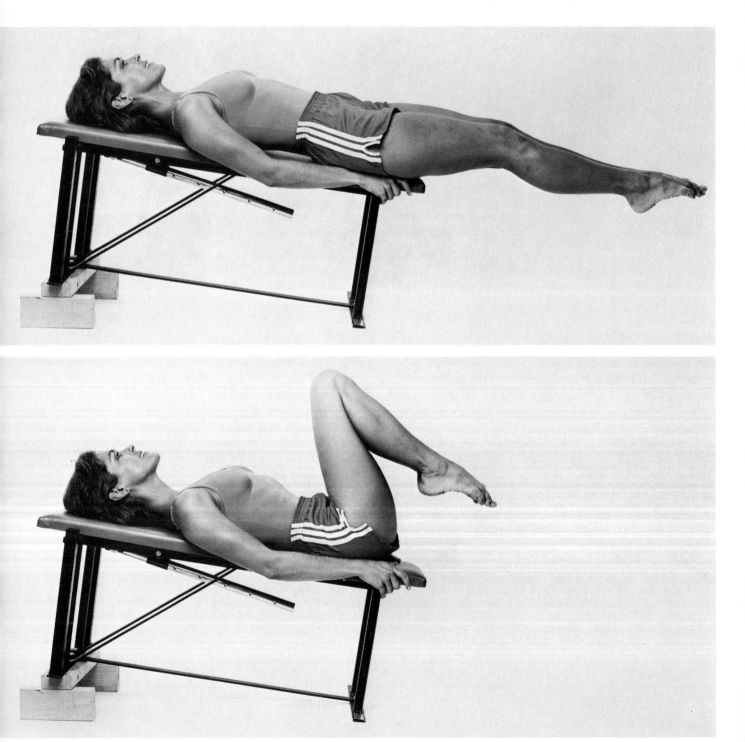

Here is your Day-30 program which will be followed on Days 30, 33, 37, 40, 44, 47, 51 and 54. These exercises will work the chest, shoulders, triceps and abdominal muscles.

EXERCISE	Page	First Level	Middle Level	Top Level
Push-ups (warm-up)	100	1 set, 12 reps	1 set, 12 reps	1 set, 12 reps
Bench Press	101	1 set, 10 reps	2 sets, 8 reps	3 sets, 12 reps
Doorway Stretch	102	10 seconds	2 sets, 15 sec	3 sets, 20 sec
Dumbbell Fly	103	1 set, 10 reps	2 sets, 8 reps	3 sets, 12 reps
Incline Stretch Between Chairs	104	10 seconds	2 sets, 15 sec	3 sets, 20 sec
Dumbbell Press	105	1 set, 10 reps	2 sets, 8 reps	3 sets, 12 reps
One-Arm Shoulder Stretch	106	10 seconds	2 sets, 15 sec	3 sets, 20 sec
Dumbbell Side Raise	107	1 set, 10 reps	2 sets, 8 reps	3 sets, 12 reps
Doorway Isometric Lateral Stretch	108	10 seconds	2 sets, 15 sec	3 sets, 20 sec
Dumbbell Rear Raise	109	1 set, 10 reps	2 sets, 8 reps	3 sets, 12 reps
Doorway Isometric Front Stretch	110	10 seconds	2 sets, 15 sec	3 sets, 20 sec
Close-Grip Bench Press	111	1 set, 10 reps	2 sets, 8 reps	3 sets, 12 reps
Reverse Dip Between Chairs	112	10 seconds	2 sets, 15 sec	3 sets, 20 sec
Two-Arm Dumbbell Extension	113	1 set, 10 reps	2 sets, 8 reps	3 sets, 12 reps
Arms-Backward Stretch	114	10 seconds	2 sets, 15 sec	3 sets, 20 sec
Incline Knee-in	114	1 set, 20 reps	2 sets, 25 reps	3 sets, 30 reps
Bent-Leg Partial Sit-up	115	1 set, 20 reps	2 sets, 25 reps	3 sets, 30 reps

PUSH-UPS

Be sure to warm up the chest, shoulders, and triceps muscles by doing one set of Push-ups before you begin your exercises.

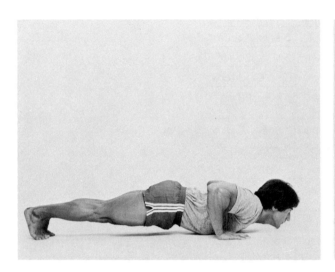
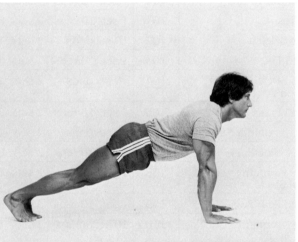
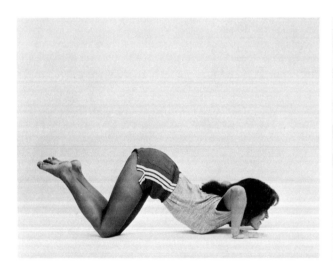
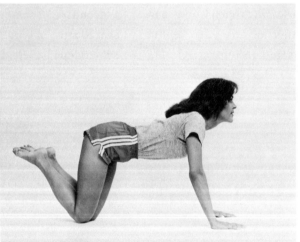

BENCH PRESS

First level: 1 set, 10 reps
Middle level: 2 sets, 8 reps
Top level: 3 sets, 12 reps

This exercise works the outer pectorals (chest) and outer deltoids when a wide grip is taken. A wide grip is harder on the shoulders, so be careful if your shoulders are sore. You can also use more weight with a wide grip because you don't have to push the weight as far. A narrower grip on the bar works more central pectoral, frontal deltoids and triceps. You will become even stronger if you lower the barbell slowly to your chest (4 seconds) and push it up a little faster (2 seconds). Your chest, shoulders and triceps will get even more pumped doing your Bench Press this way.

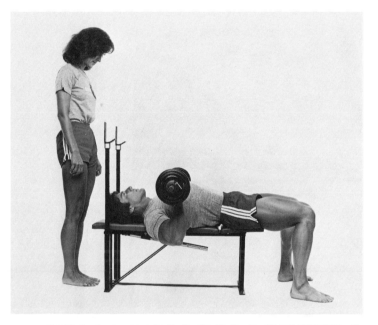

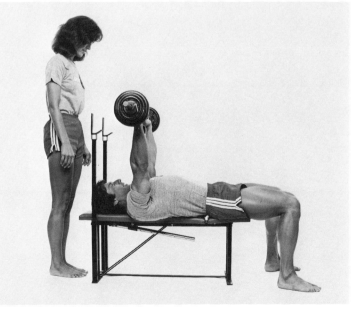

DOORWAY STRETCH

First level: 1 set, 10 sec
Middle level: 2 sets, 15 sec
Top level: 3 sets, 20 sec

This exercise gives a good stretch to the same area as Bench Press. Your flexibility has improved in this part of your body, and you'll be feeling even greater circulation in your chest and shoulders as you continue.

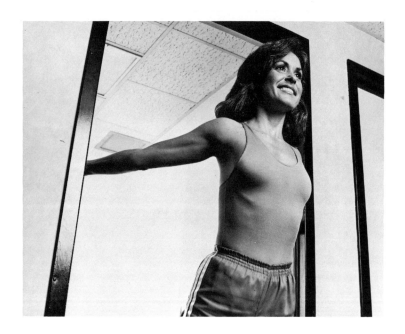

DUMBBELL FLY

First level: 1 set, 10 reps
Middle level: 2 sets, 8 reps
Top level: 3 sets, 12 reps

Lie on a flat bench with your feet flat on the floor at each side of the bench, or with your knees bent and feet flat on the end of the bench. Hold a dumbbell in each hand, over your chest, with your elbows slightly bent. Keep your elbows in this position as you inhale and extend your arms out to each side until the dumbbells are level or slightly lower than the level of the bench. Exhale as you slowly bring the dumbbells back over your chest. Repeat.

This is probably the single best exercise for developing the outer pectorals. By stretching down to the sides as far as possible, you bring the outer pecs strongly into action, and your chest will feel expanded. Immediately after Dumbbell Fly do Incline Stretch Between Chairs.

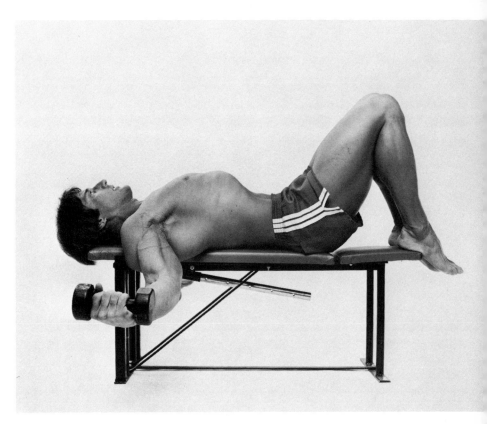

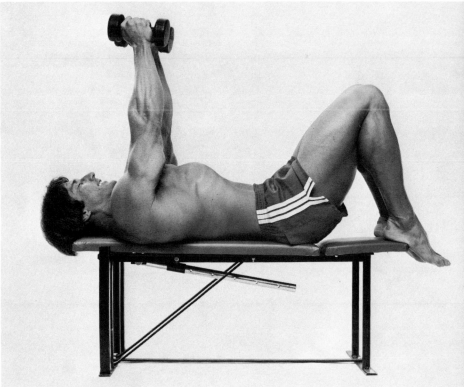

103

INCLINE STRETCH BETWEEN CHAIRS

First level: 1 set, 10 sec
Middle level: 2 sets, 15 sec
Top level: 3 sets, 20 sec

Assume push-up position with your toes touching the floor and each hand on a chair seat, placed slightly wider than your shoulders. Lower to the bottom position and hold for the designated time.

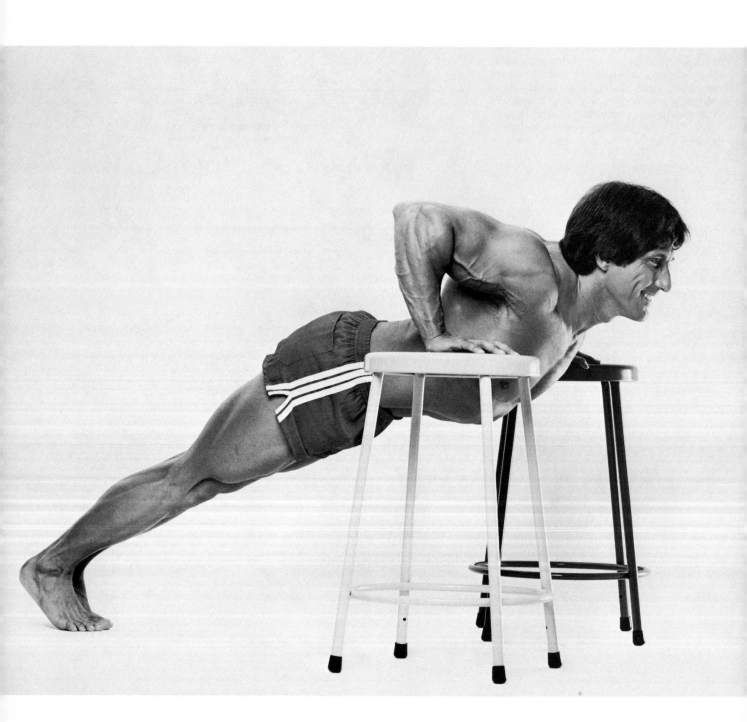

104

DUMBBELL PRESS

First level: 1 set, 10 reps
Middle level: 2 sets, 8 reps
Top level: 3 sets, 12 reps

This exercise not only works all three sections of the shoulder muscles (front, side and rear deltoids) when the dumbbells are pressed up and lowered in a straight line parallel to the neck, but also works the upper chest and triceps. It is a good substitute for the Press Behind Neck. Stand or sit erect. Hold one dumbbell in each hand at shoulder level, out to each side of your shoulders. Have the dumbbells face each other, end to end. Exhale as you press the dumbbells overhead, where they will touch ends. Inhale and slowly lower the dumbbells back to each side of your shoulders.

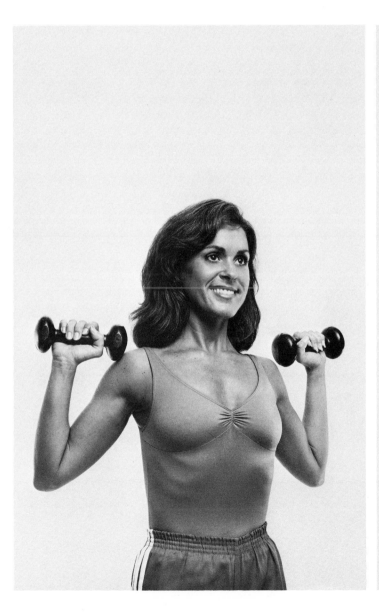
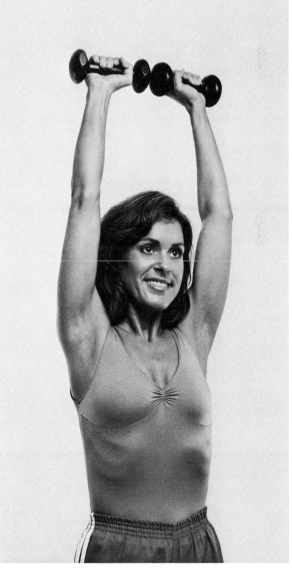

ONE-ARM SHOULDER STRETCH

First level: 1 set, 10 sec
Middle level: 2 sets, 15 sec
Top level: 3 sets, 20 sec

Do this stretch the same way you did it in the Basic Program. You'll feel even more stimulation in the shoulders when you do One-Arm Shoulder Stretch immediately after the Dumbbell Press. Gradually increase the resistance by pulling a little harder as you hold for the designated time.

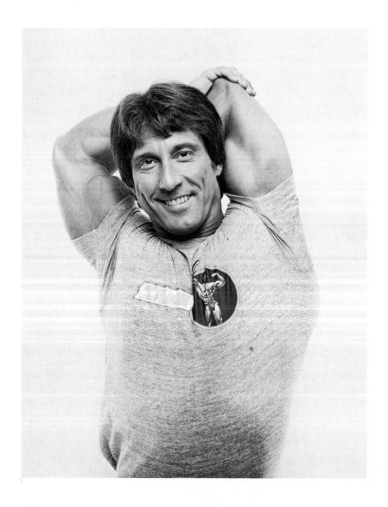

DUMBBELL SIDE RAISE

First level: 1 set, 10 reps
Middle level: 2 sets, 8 reps
Top level: 3 sets, 12 reps

This new exercise and stretch directly affects the side or lateral deltoids. Stand or sit and hold a dumbbell in each hand, down at your sides. Inhale as you slowly raise the dumbbells above shoulder level keeping your arms straight and turning the backs of the dumbbells slightly up. Pause momentarily. Exhale as you slowly lower the dumbbells back to your sides. This exercise develops the side or lateral deltoid and adds width to the shoulders. Do the movement slowly and feel your deltoids expanding.

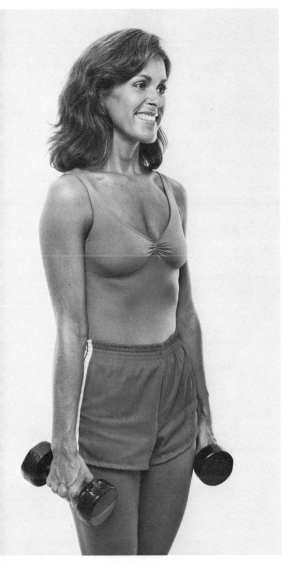
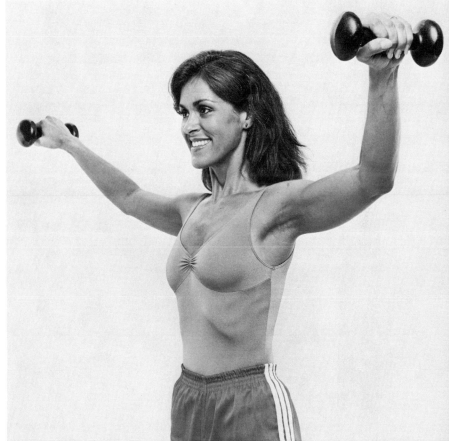

107

DOORWAY ISOMETRIC LATERAL STRETCH

First level: 1 set, 10 sec
Middle level: 2 sets, 15 sec
Top level: 3 sets, 20 sec

Stand inside a doorway, holding your arms straight down to each side and making fists with each hand. Extend your arms until they contact the doorway and press against it, gradually increasing the tension until the designated time is up. When you finish you will feel the blood circulating through the side deltoids.

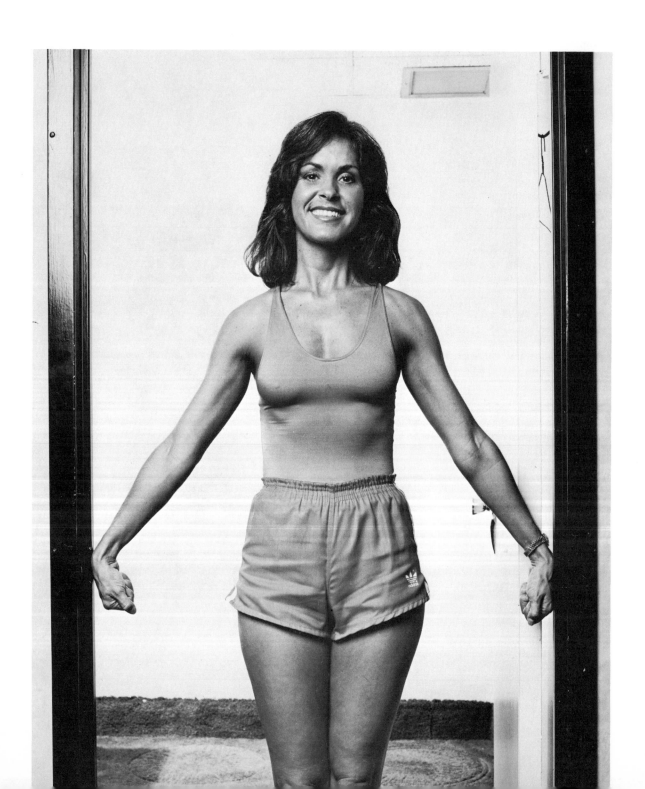

DUMBBELL REAR RAISE

First level: 1 set, 10 reps
Middle level: 2 sets, 8 reps
Top level: 3 sets, 12 reps

This exercise will thoroughly work the rear deltoids, which is a relatively difficult area to reach. Stand, bent over at the waist, with your knees slightly bent. Hold a dumbbell in each hand, with your arms extended straight down to the floor. Inhale as you raise the dumbbells out to each side, with straight arms, and the backs of the wrists turned slightly upward, until they are above the level of your back. Exhale as you slowly lower the dumbbells until your hands meet. Stay bent over and repeat. This exercise adds a squared-off broad look to your shoulders. You'll feel the pump in your upper back and the backs of your shoulders.

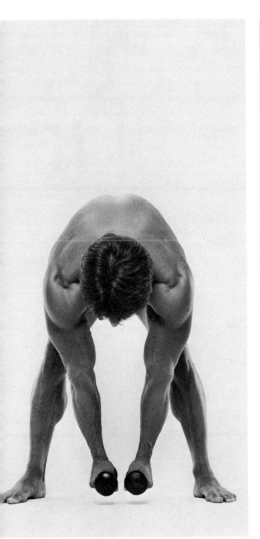

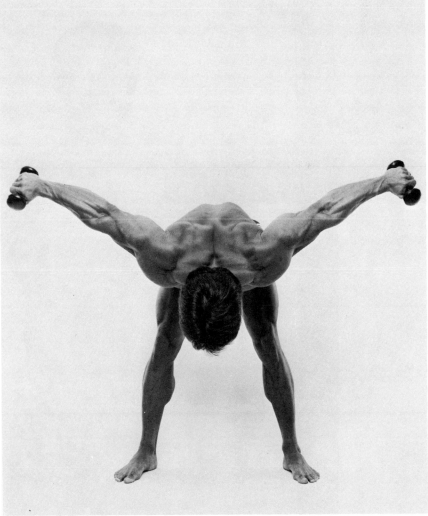

109

DOORWAY ISOMETRIC
FRONT STRETCH

First level: 1 set, 10 sec
Middle level: 2 sets, 15 sec
Top level: 3 sets, 20 sec

Stand at arms' distance from and facing an open doorway. Bring your arms up to chest level, extended to the front, and make a fist with each hand. Spread open your arms until they touch the inside of the doorjamb. Press your fists and wrists against the doorjamb, tensing your chest, back and shoulders. Hold this tension for the designated time and then relax. This will stretch and develop as well as strengthen your side and rear deltoids. Feel them working deeply.

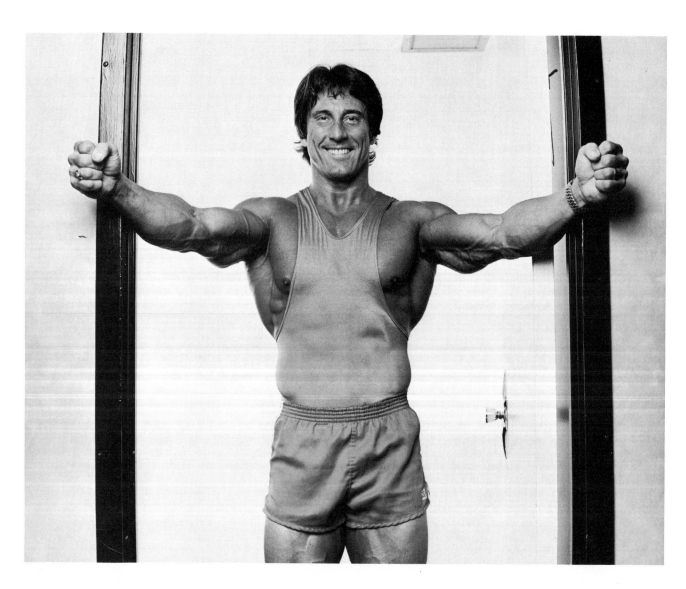

CLOSE-GRIP BENCH PRESS

First level: 1 set, 10 reps
Middle level: 2 sets, 8 reps
Top level: 3 sets, 12 reps

Do this movement as you have been doing it before. Concentrate on your outer triceps and feel this exercise working them with each repetition. The more you keep your elbows out to the side, the more you will feel the effects in the outer triceps. Be sure to lower the bar slowly. Immediately after this exercise do Reverse Dip Between Chairs.

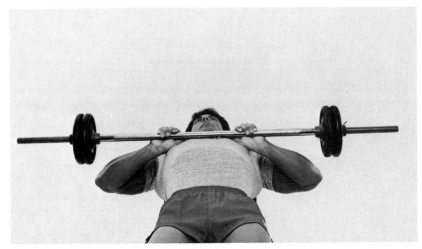

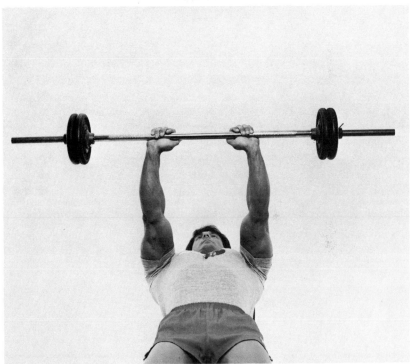

111

REVERSE DIP BETWEEN CHAIRS

First level: 1 set, 10 sec
Middle level: 2 sets, 15 sec
Top level: 3 sets, 20 sec

Place two chairs side by side at the width of your shoulders. Stand in front of the chairs, squat down and place the palms of your hands, with your fingers pointing forward, on the chairs. Extend your legs straight out in front of you, with your feet together and your knees straight. Begin with your elbows straight. Slowly inhale as you lower yourself below the level of the seats of the chairs. Hold this stretch. You will feel it in the triceps and rear deltoid muscles.

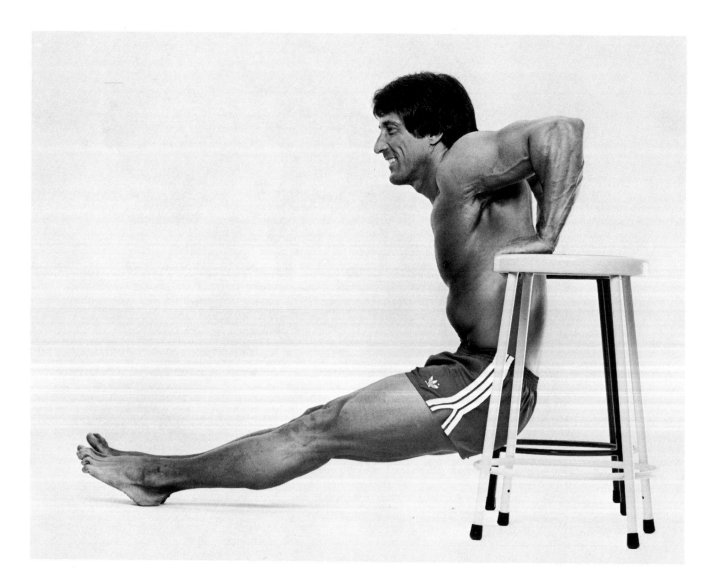

112

TWO-ARM DUMBBELL EXTENSION

First level: 1 set, 10 reps
Middle level: 2 sets, 8 reps
Top level: 3 sets, 12 reps

This is a new exercise in your Intermediate Program. Stand or sit, holding a dumbbell with both hands by hooking your thumbs around the bar and allowing the plate to rest on your open hands with the palms facing upward. Bring the dumbbell above your head. Your arms should be pulled back so that your elbows are very close in toward your ears. Hold your arms in this position and inhale as you lower the dumbbell until your arms are fully bent. Exhale as you press the dumbbell overhead until your elbows are nearly straight. This exercise is an all-around triceps developer. Feel the stretch as you lower the dumbbell behind your head as low as it will go. Tense your triceps hard as your elbows lock out.

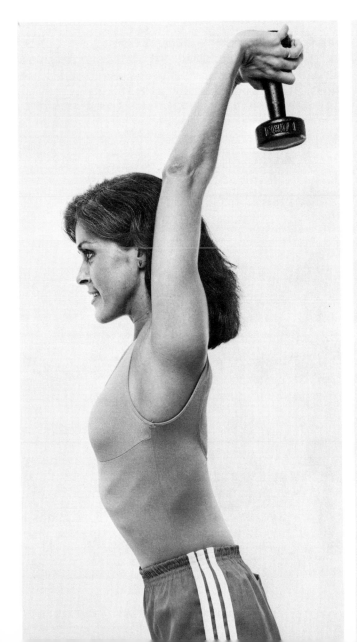
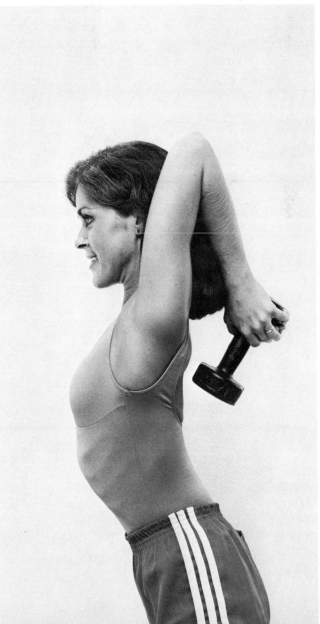

ARMS-BACKWARD STRETCH

First level: 1 set, 10 sec
Middle level: 2 sets, 15 sec
Top level: 3 sets, 20 sec

INCLINE KNEE-IN

First level: 1 set, 20 reps
Middle level: 2 sets, 25 reps
Top level: 3 sets, 30 reps

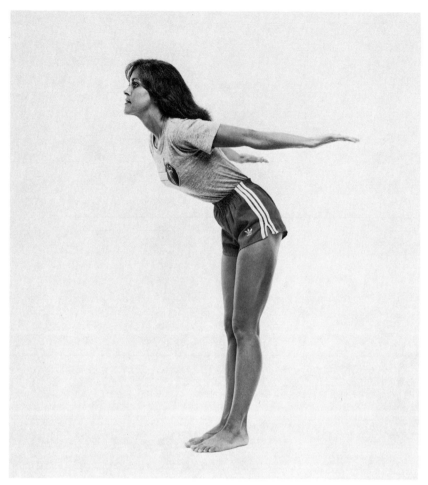

Do this exercise immediately following Two-Arm Dumbbell Extension. You've done this before; but this time try to get the maximum possible stretch by tensing the triceps and the rear deltoids. Feel the stimulation in these areas. Now do Incline Knee-in.

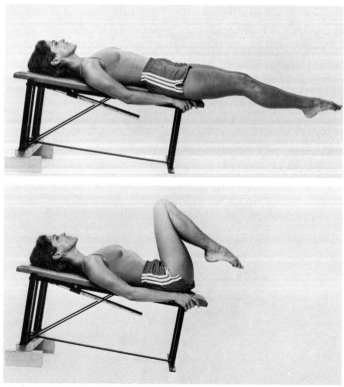

BENT-LEG PARTIAL SIT-UP

First level: 1 set, 20 reps
Middle level: 2 sets, 25 reps
Top level: 3 sets, 30 reps

A lot of people think that the best exercise for the waistline is the sit-ups. Actually Sit-ups only work the abdominals through a small portion of the sitting-up motion and work the lower-back area the rest of the time. We prefer Bent-Leg Partial Sit-up because the abdominals are given concentrated work. Do these as you did them in the Basic Program, but with one slight modification: At the point where your head, shoulders and hips are thrust into their highest position, tense the abdominals and hold for a count of two. Do all the repetitions this way.

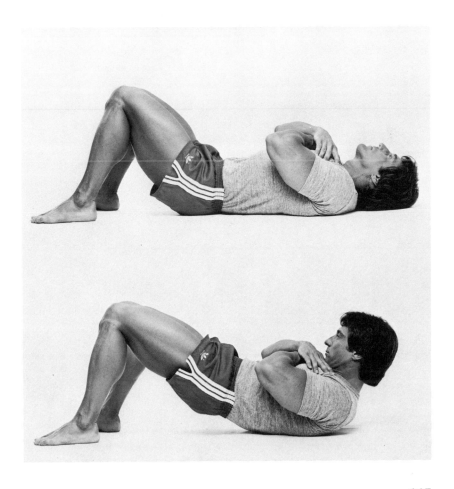

115

Here is your Day-31 program which will be used on Days 31, 34, 38, 41, 45, 48, 52 and 55. These exercises will work the muscles of your lower body.

EXERCISE	Page	First Level	Middle Level	Top Level
One-Leg Top Extension (warm-up)	117	1 set, 25 reps	1 set, 25 reps	1 set, 25 reps
Half Squat	118	1 set, 12 reps	2 sets, 8 reps	3 sets, 15 reps
Lunge with Back Foot on Bench	119	10 seconds	2 sets, 15 sec	3 sets, 20 sec
Hack Squat	120	1 set, 10 reps	2 sets, 8 reps	3 sets, 12 reps
Forward Stretch	121	10 seconds	2 sets, 15 sec	3 sets, 20 sec
Stiff-Legged Deadlift	122	1 set, 10 reps	2 sets, 8 reps	3 sets, 12 reps
One-Leg-up Stretch	123	10 seconds	2 sets, 15 sec	3 sets, 20 sec
Donkey Calf Raise	124	1 set, 25 reps	2 sets, 20 reps	3 sets, 25 reps
Two-Leg Calf Stretch	124	10 seconds	2 sets, 15 sec	3 sets, 20 sec
One-Leg Calf Raise	125	1 set, 12 reps	2 sets, 15 reps	3 sets, 15 reps
Wall Lean (for calves)	126	10 seconds	2 sets, 15 sec	3 sets, 20 sec
Incline Knee-in	127	1 set, 20 reps	2 sets, 25 reps	3 sets, 30 reps
Bent-Leg Partial Sit-up	128	1 set, 20 reps	2 sets, 25 reps	3 sets, 30 reps
Seated Twist	129	1 set, 20 reps	2 sets, 25 reps	3 sets, 30 reps

ONE-LEG TOP EXTENSION

You've been doing this exercise for the past 4 weeks, so you are aware of the warming-up and loosening effect it has on the knees. In the Intermediate Program go up to 25 reps for one set before you begin the Half Squat.

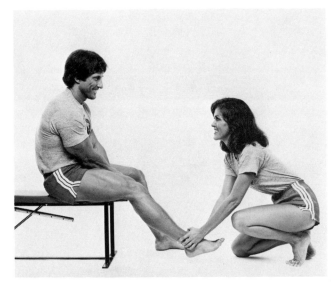

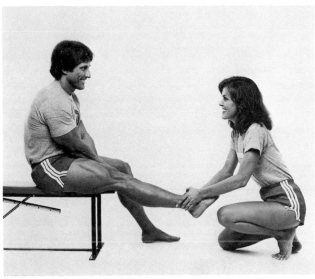

HALF SQUAT

First level: 1 set, 10 reps
Middle level: 2 sets, 8 reps
Top level: 3 sets, 12 reps

You will be doing more repetitions on Half Squat than you did in the Basic Program, which will further stimulate deep breathing as well as your thigh development. Do each repetition slowly, especially when descending to the bench, and come up a little faster (4 seconds down, 2 seconds up). You will feel a greater pump in the thighs doing them this way, and your lower back will become stronger, too.

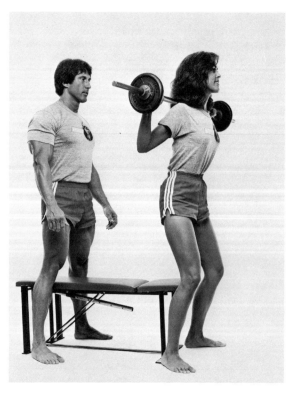 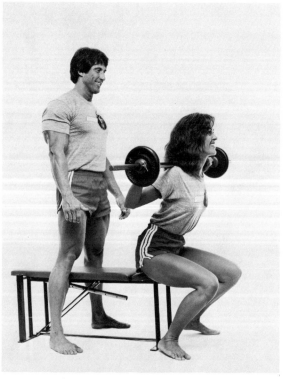

118

LUNGE WITH BACK FOOT ON BENCH

First level: 1 set, 10 sec
Middle level: 2 sets, 15 sec
Top level: 3 sets, 20 sec

You've been doing this stretch for the last 4 weeks in the Basic Program, and it is continued into the Intermediate Program. Lunge even more deeply than you have in the past. The deeper you go, the more you will feel the stretch in your thighs and buttocks. Be extra careful to slowly descend into the deep lunge position before you begin holding for the designated time.

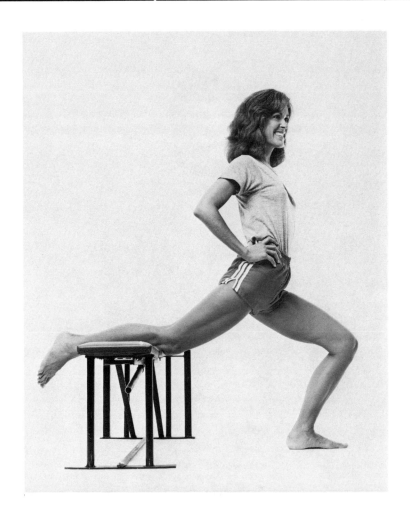

HACK SQUAT

First level: 1 set, 10 reps
Middle level: 2 sets, 8 reps
Top level: 3 sets, 12 reps

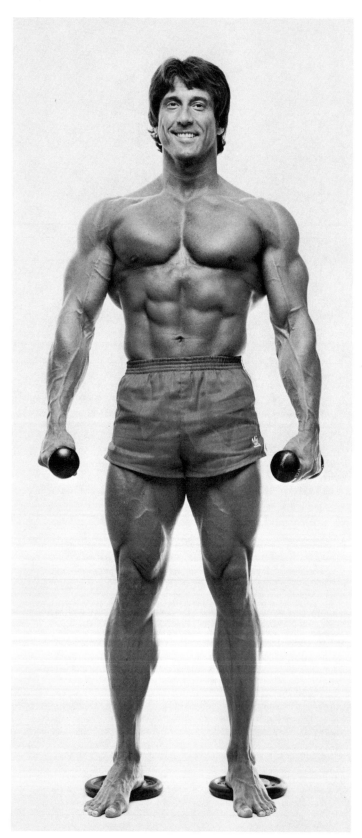

This is a great exercise for the thighs, especially when done following Half Squat and Lunge with Back Foot on Bench. Stand with a dumbbell in each hand and with a board about ¾ inch thick under your heels. Keep your back straight and your hips forward as you slowly lower to a parallel squat position, inhaling as you go down. Exhale as you slowly rise up, bringing your hips forward and keeping your back straight until you're standing upright again. Repeat this exercise; you will feel the frontal thigh muscles expand, especially the area right above the knees.

Be sure to lower as far as possible in the squat for maximum effect. This is a new exercise in your Intermediate Program, and you will feel it more and more as you perfect your form in the movement.

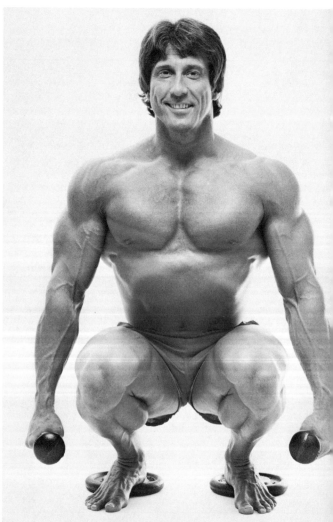

FORWARD STRETCH

First level: 1 set, 10 sec
Middle level: 2 sets, 15 sec
Top level: 3 sets, 20 sec

This should be done just as you did it in the Basic Program. By now, however, your lower back and the backs of your thighs and buttocks have loosened up and you'll be able to go down a little farther with your hands than you did when you started. Keep your knees bent if you feel a strain in the lower back area or if you've had problems there before.

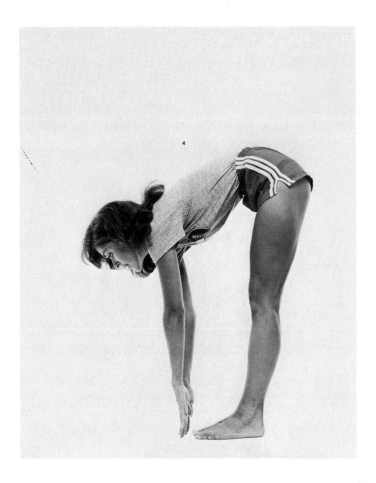

STIFF-LEGGED DEADLIFT

First level: 1 set, 10 reps
Middle level: 2 sets, 8 reps
Top level: 3 sets, 12 reps

The following are two of the best exercises for stretching the leg biceps (hamstrings), buttocks and lower back.

Stand with your feet 6 inches apart, holding a barbell in your hands where it crosses your thighs, while your arms are held straight down. If you are very flexible, you may wish to stand on a block to get an even better stretch. Inhale and bend over at the waist, keeping your knees straight, until the barbell touches the floor, or you reach maximum stretch. Exhale and return slowly to standing position.

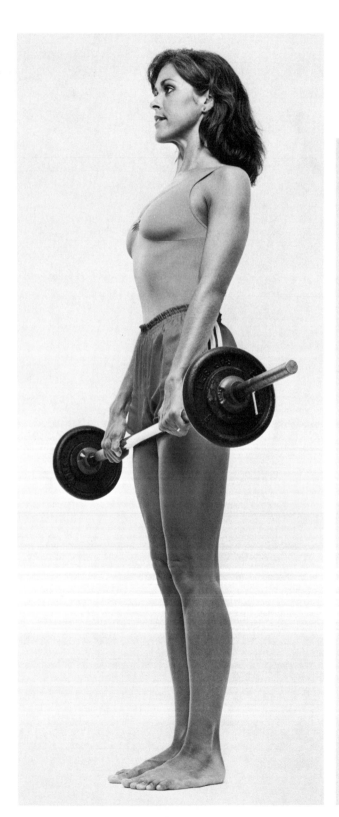
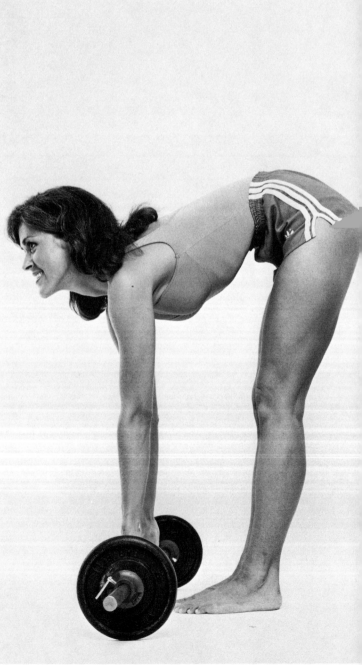

ONE-LEG-UP STRETCH

First level: 1 set, 10 sec
Middle level: 2 sets, 15 sec
Top level: 3 sets, 20 sec

Stand leg distance from a table, or ballet barre which is at least waist high. Lift one leg while keeping the other straight and rest it on the ballet barre or table. Do not bend your knees. Stretch forward toward the toes of the raised leg and hold for the designated time. Relax. Switch to stretch the other leg. Working one leg at a time gives a more concentrated stretch in the rear thigh, hips and lower back.

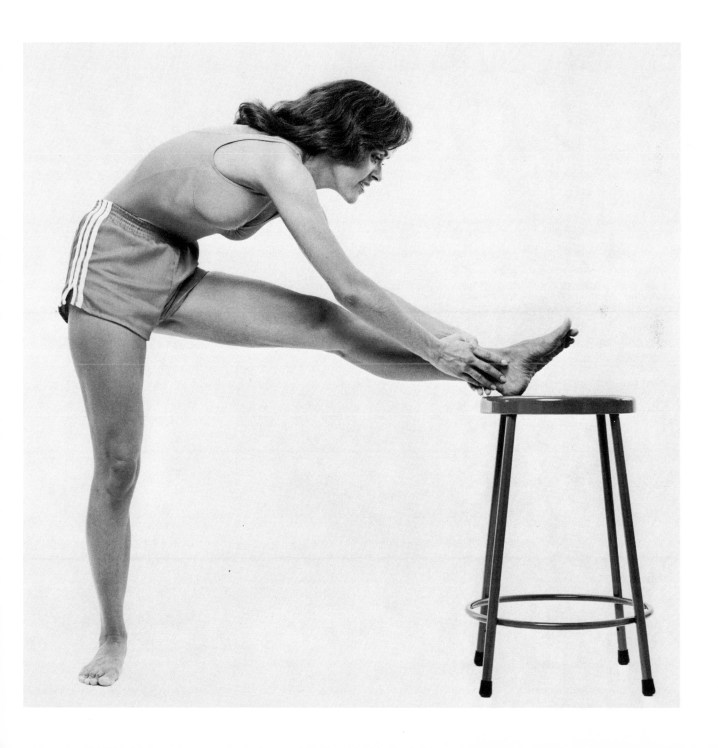

DONKEY CALF RAISE

First level: 1 set, 20 reps
Middle level: 2 sets, 15 reps
Top level: 3 sets, 25 reps

TWO-LEG CALF STRETCH

First level: 1 set, 10 sec
Middle level: 2 sets, 15 sec
Top level: 3 sets, 20 sec

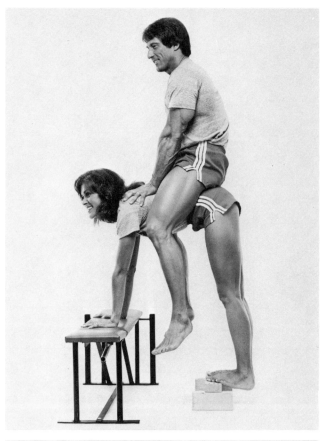

Do these just as you did in the Basic Program. Are you doing them with your knees bent or straight? Both ways are okay, and you can interchange them for variation. Keeping the knees bent will give more of a stretch and develop the lower part of your calf. Doing them with your knees locked will develop and stretch the area right below the back of your knees (upper calf).

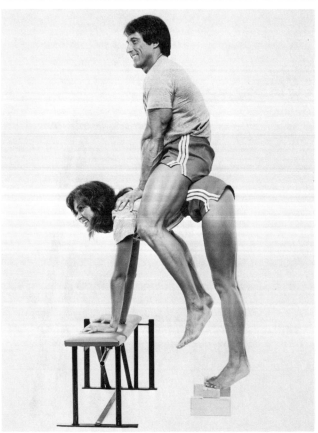

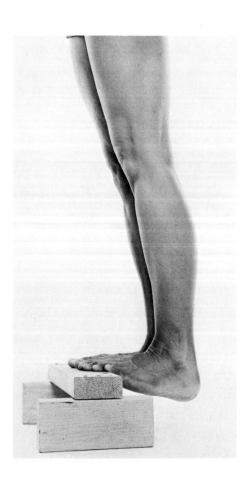

First level: 1 set, 12 reps
Middle level: 2 sets, 15 reps
Top level: 3 sets, 15 reps

ONE-LEG CALF RAISE

This is a difficult exercise to do, so the repetitions listed are lower. You may also find that one leg is stronger than the other. By practicing it you will eventually be able to balance the calf strength in each leg. To do this exercise stand on a calf block with one foot, toes resting on the block. Lift the other leg, with the knee bent, and either hold it in midair or rest it on the back of the opposite leg's knee. Slowly raise high and lower very deeply on your toes. Do this movement on both legs. One-Leg Calf Raise works the outer calf if the toes are pointed in and the inner calf if the toes are pointed out (provided you keep your balance on the ball of your foot and the first two toes). It is very good for strengthening the ankles. Descend as far as possible for a maximum pump and stretch in the lower calf.

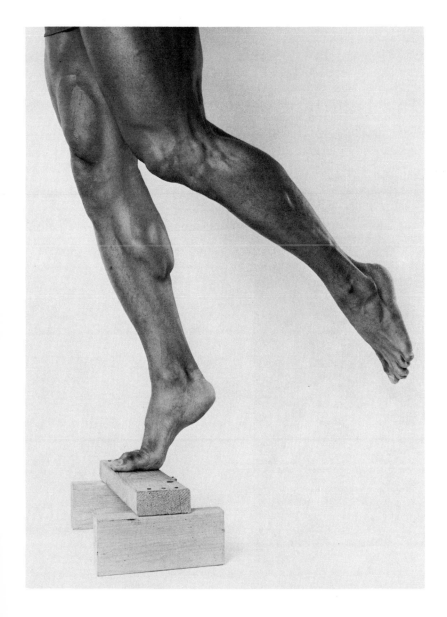

WALL LEAN

First level: 1 set, 10 sec
Middle level: 2 sets, 15 sec
Top level: 3 sets, 20 sec

Do this stretch by standing out a little farther from the wall compared to the way you did it on Day 29. This stretch works the calves and forearms. Concentrate on stretching your calves and feel the effects very deeply in this area.

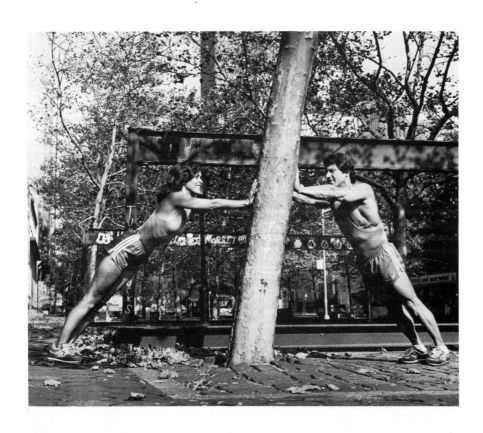

INCLINE KNEE-IN

First level: 1 set, 20 reps
Middle level: 2 sets, 25 reps
Top level: 3 sets, 30 reps

Prop a flat bench up on your calf block to form an incline. Lie on the safely secured bench and do the exercise in the same way that you did the Flat Knee-in during the Basic Program. This exercise tightens the lower abdominal area at the navel and below—a part of the body where fat accumulates easily. Keep your abdominals flexed as you do each repetition.

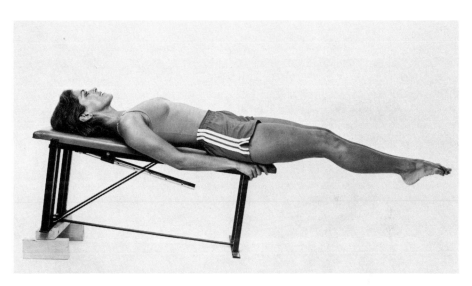

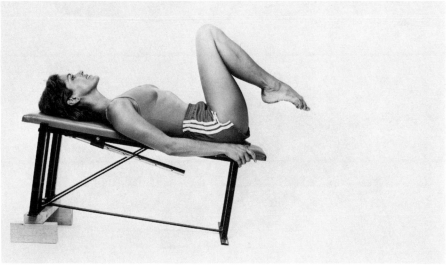

127

BENT-LEG PARTIAL SIT-UP

First level: 1 set, 20 reps
Middle level: 2 sets, 25 reps
Top level: 3 sets, 30 reps

A lot of people think that the best exercise for their waistline is Sit-ups. Actually the lower back does most of the work in Sit-ups, and the abdominals are used only through a small portion of the sitting-up motion. We prefer Bent-Leg Partial Sit-up because only the abdominals are given concentrated work. Do these as you did in the Basic Program, but with one slight modification: At the point where your head, shoulders and hips are thrust into their highest position, tense the abdominals and hold on for a count of two. Do all your reps in this manner.

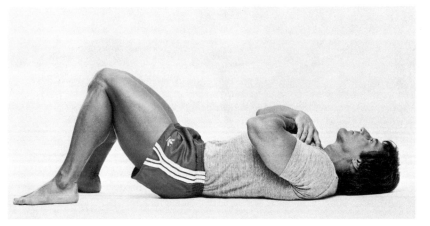

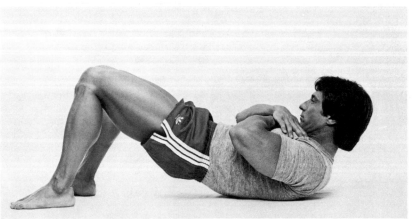

SEATED TWIST

First level: 1 set, 20 reps
Middle level: 2 sets, 25 reps
Top level: 3 sets, 30 reps

This is the best exercise we have found for trimming the sides of the waist (external oblique muscles) and the lower back, eliminating the "spare tire" look. You've been doing this exercise since the Basic Program and if the designated number of repetitions is too easy for you now, then try doing the total number of reps in one set. For example, instead of doing 2 sets of 25 reps, do 1 set of 50 reps. If you're following the first level of the program, increase the number of reps you do for the 1 set. Increases by tens are the best way to do this. Remember always to begin twisting slowly and gradually increase the speed.

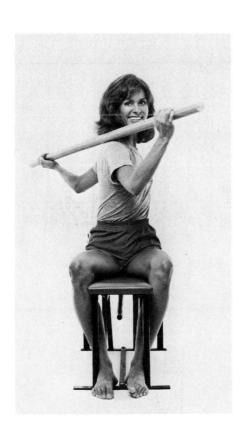

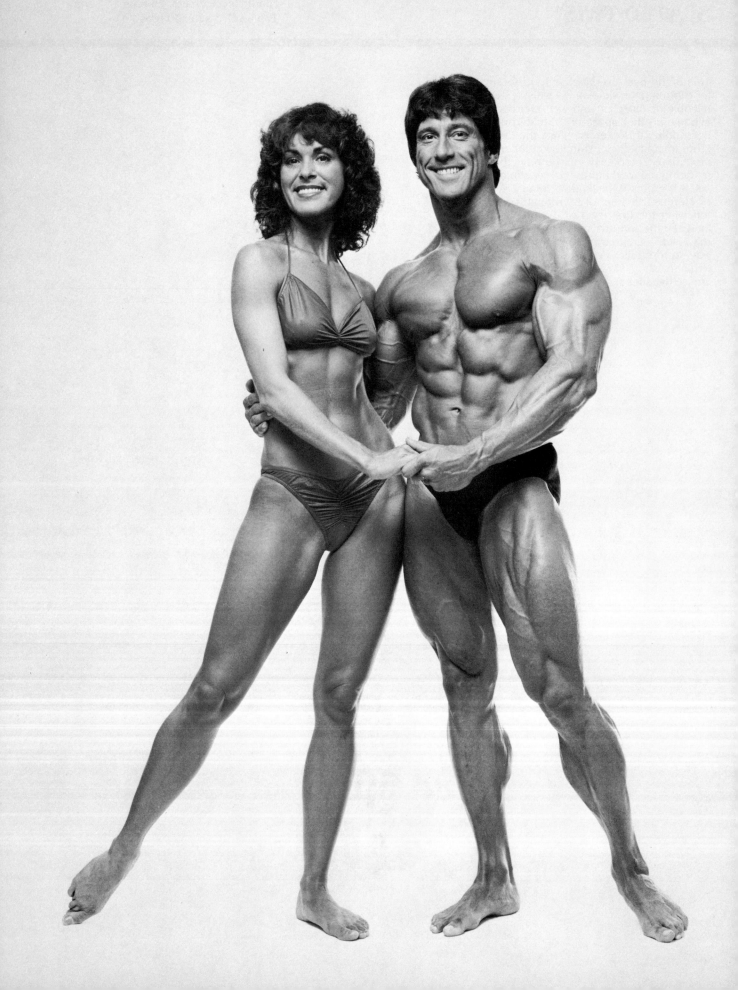

DAILY INTERMEDIATE PROGRAM
Weeks 5 to 8

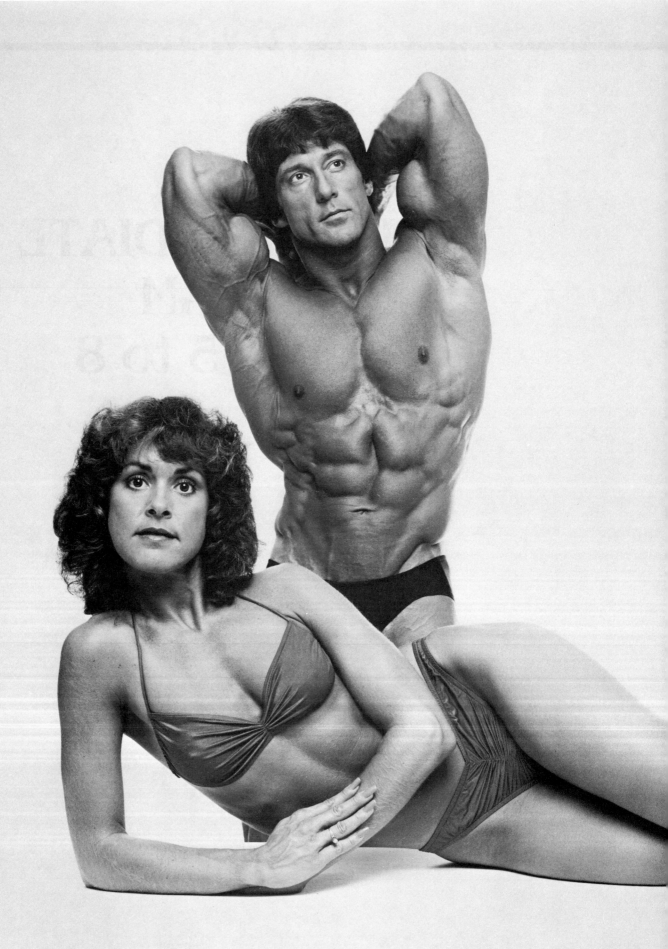

Week Five
Day 29

AEROBIC EXERCISES

Check the Basic Program, Day 1, to review the form of Quick Paced Step-ups. You should be able to begin at a fairly quick pace after warming up, and keep it there. Get your knees high on each Step-up. This will work the rear of the thigh as well as the buttocks. After you have made certain that your step or bench is solid and doesn't move or wobble, set your timer for 2 minutes; take a deep breath; exhale completely and begin. When you are finished you will need more time to warm down than previously.

WEIGHT TRAINING AND STRETCHING

The Day-29 program works back, biceps, forearms and abdominal muscles. All the new exercises have been explained. If you have been doing an exercise in the Basic Program and are continuing into the Intermediate Program, we'll give you some further instruction; but do remember to continue at the same level (First, Middle, Top) that you followed in the Basic Program. If you don't fully understand the exercise and how to do it correctly, don't hesitate to refer to the photos or descriptions elsewhere in the book.

INTERMEDIATE DIET TIPS

Continue to note in your food record the type and amounts of food that you eat. In the Intermediate Program you will be moving toward a diet more closely personalized to your specific needs and goals. If you still need to eliminate and substitute foods, then continue doing so for as long as necessary. We suggest that you begin dropping more of the extremely high carbohydrate foods and substituting for them foods that are lower in carbohydrates yet high in nutrition. We have given some recipes in the recipe section, which should help you make your choices.

Begin to control the amount of food that you eat as well as the times when you eat. Remember, you don't need as many calories or carbohydrates late in the day as you do in the morning. When planning your menus, consider what your physical output will be during the day.

We will give you specific menus and recipes to either trim or build your body. Begin thinking about the direction that you would like to take, and discuss this in your household and/or with your training partner. Being aware of the needs of those around you can enable you to provide support for their goals; and in return they can do the same for you. Everyone benefits from encouragement.

Day 30

AEROBIC EXERCISE

Set your timer for 2 minutes and 15 seconds for Quick Paced Step-ups. Take a deep breath, exhale totally and begin. Lift your knees high and swing your arms gently. You should be feeling this in the front of your thighs and in your buttocks.

WEIGHT TRAINING AND STRETCHING

Today you will exercise the pushing muscles of the upper body—chest, shoulders and triceps—as well as your waistline. Stay at the same level as in the Basic Program (First, Middle or Top). Be sure to look up the directions, photographs and descriptions of those exercises that you are not sure of.

Day 31

AEROBIC EXERCISE

Set your timer for 2 minutes and 30 seconds for the Quick Paced Step-ups. Keep your pace regular and quick from start to finish. Walk around slowly afterward to bring your breathing back to normal.

WEIGHT TRAINING AND STRETCHING

Today you will begin exercising your legs and waist. This program is slightly longer and progressively more difficult than the Basic leg program. Continue at the same level as in the Basic Program.

Day 32

AEROBIC EXERCISE

Two minutes and 45 seconds is the total time for Quick Paced Step-ups today. You should have no trouble handling the 15-second increase. Your endurance and stamina just keep improving.

WEIGHT TRAINING AND STRETCHING

Today you will repeat the Day-29 program, exercising and stretching the pulling muscles of the upper body, as well as the abdominals. You should be fully rested in these areas because the last time you worked the pulling muscles was three days ago. You will begin to notice that you have more strength when you work each part twice a week as opposed to three times a week in the Basic Program.

Day 33

AEROBIC EXERCISE

Today your Quick Paced Step-ups will be done for 3 minutes. Keep a fast pace. If you have good form in the exercise it will be easier to do for longer periods of time. Set your timer and begin.

WEIGHT TRAINING AND STRETCHING

Repeat Day 30 and really work the pushing muscles of your upper body! Remember that your goal is to keep your rest periods between sets to 1½ to 2 minutes. If you time how long it takes for your breathing to return to normal it should be approximately this amount of time. Keep your pace up throughout the entire workout and continue to encourage your partner.

Day 34

AEROBIC EXERCISE

Yesterday's aerobics were easier than before, and the same will be true today. Set your timer for 3 minutes and 15 seconds. Think in a positive way about all the improvements you're making and about how wonderful you look and feel. Give more today than you ever have before. Be happy about yourself and your exercise program. The time will fly by! Use the proper amount of time to cool off and relax.

WEIGHT TRAINING AND STRETCHING

Today you will exercise your lower body using the Day-31 program. This is your fifth week of exercise, and the changes in the way you look and feel are becoming more and more evident to both you and others. To continue making these improvements you should keep feeling the effects of your workouts. When you train you should experience a pump in the muscles being worked. Immediately after your workout you should feel totally exhilarated from the increased amount of circulation that the weight training and stretching have induced. Several hours following your workout you should feel pleasantly tired in the exercised area. Ideally this sensation should occur right before bedtime and serve as a natural tranquilizer. This is your last day of exercise for Week 5, so go and do your very best!

Day 35

AEROBIC EXERCISE, WEIGHT TRAINING AND STRETCHING

This is your well-earned day of rest. Was this first week of the Intermediate Program easier or more difficult for you than Week 4 of the Basic Program? If you found it easier, then try resting slightly less between sets and/or using a little more weight. Because each body part is worked from more angles, the Intermediate Program uses more exercises for each part of the body and helps you develop a better shape to your muscles.

MUTUAL-ASSISTANCE TECHNIQUE

Are you and your partner moving through your workout without wasting time? Do you sit around and talk between sets? Distractions will prevent you from getting a better workout. When you're doing a set, your partner should protect you from distracting influences and vice versa. When you are doing your set, your job is to do the best you possibly can. What distracts you? Are there any ways in which you and your partner can minimize these distractions?

BODY AWARENESS

Take a set of "before" photographs to be placed in your records for reference. The photos should be well lit so that you can see every area of your body clearly. Take a photo of your partner, and have your partner take one of you in the following four poses:

1. Standing relaxed, feet 2 to 3 inches apart, arms down to your sides, facing forward.
2. Standing the same way as the first pose, facing to the right side.
3. Again same as the first pose, this time facing to the left.
4. Turn around, stand the same way you did in pose 1 to take a photo of your back side.

You should take these photos in the nude or with as little on as possible. It's helpful to take color and black-and-white photos, as well as color slides. Have 8-by-10 photos developed and include them in your record as soon as possible. You will be using them to pinpoint the changes that you would like to see in your body later in the program. Put a date and the word *before* on these photos.

Create a section in your journal for keeping notes on the Body Awareness exercises you will be doing. Always date each entry. Keep your "before" photos here also. Write down a list of all the changes you wish to see in your body at the end of the 12-week period. Be specific. Write them down in the sequence in which they come to you. When you have finished, read over the changes and begin visualizing them as having already taken place.

Week Six
Day 36

AEROBIC EXERCISE

High Kicks is your exercise for this week. You will be able to kick your legs higher and will find it easier and easier as the week progresses. You will notice that your abdomen will become firmer—especially the lower abdomen—and that there will be fewer and fewer wrinkles around the top of your leg biceps and at the base of your buttocks. As you lift your leg, tighten your buttocks and pull your stomach in. Concentrate on working these areas and on keeping up a quick pace. If you don't remember the specifics, read over the Aerobics section for Week 2—Days 8 through 14—before you set your timer for 2 minutes. Take the proper warm-down time after the exercise.

WEIGHT TRAINING AND STRETCHING

Today you feel strong and refreshed after yesterday's rest. Repeat Day 29 and exercise the pulling muscles of the upper body. This will be the third time you have done this workout, and today it will be easier than ever before. Rest only long enough between sets to allow your breathing to return to normal before beginning the next set. With big muscle groups like back or thighs you are probably noticing that the recovery time is slightly longer than it is with smaller muscle groups like biceps and triceps. This is normal, so allow for the extra time in your workouts.

INTERMEDIATE DIET TIPS

Update and improve your record book. Make a column for the date, the time of day, your location, what you ate, the amounts that you ate, the calorie content, carbohydrate, protein and fat grams. Fill this in each time you eat.

Form a new section in your notebook for Sensory Awareness. At the end of each meal write how you feel. Write it in a sensory way. For example, try to get away from describing your feelings with adjectives like terrific, sensational, and in some cases . . . lousy. Instead, describe your bodily sensations. How do things feel inside? What tastes do you sense after eating? How do you feel psychologically? Write whatever comes to mind first, without altering it. Reread what you record often. This is the most effective way of determining for yourself what and how to eat properly. You are preparing yourself to set up your personal, lifetime program.

SUPER BODIES IN 12 WEEKS

Day 37

AEROBIC EXERCISE

Prepare yourself for doing the High Kicks by taking a deep breath and exhaling the air from your lungs completely. Then set your timer for 2 minutes, 15 seconds, and begin. When finished, take the proper time to cool down and relax.

WEIGHT TRAINING AND STRETCHING

Repeat Day 30 today for chest, shoulders, triceps and abdominal muscles. By working all these muscle groups on one day you get a very concentrated, efficient workout because just about every exercise (with the exception of those for the waist) works more than one area. Whenever you work the chest, you also work the shoulders and triceps to some extent. You also get indirect upper chest and tricep work when you do some of the shoulder exercises. Tricep work also affects the chest and shoulders to some extent. So what you have is constant stimulation for these muscle groups throughout the entire workout.

Day 38

AEROBIC EXERCISE

Concentrating on a given body part will help to work the area more effectively. We are concerned with getting more from the aerobic exercises than just the aerobic effects. Why not give the muscles all over your body a workout too? When you are doing the High Kicks do you keep your foot flexed, pushing your heel out and pulling your toes back toward your body? Put your attention on doing this today. Keep the pace going quickly and don't let up. Every day you will increase the pace just a little bit more, but never go so fast that the form of the exercise suffers. Set your timer for 2 minutes and 30 seconds and begin your High Kicks. Take the proper warm-down time following the exercise.

WEIGHT TRAINING AND STRETCHING

Today you will repeat the Day-31 program for the lower body. Do you always use a weight heavy enough to permit you to do only the designated amount of repetitions and no more? Unless you do this, the exercises will not stimulate the muscles deeply enough. Always check the poundages you used in prior workouts for the same body parts. Before you begin today, check over the poundages you used on Day 34, the last time you worked the lower body. Resolve constantly to do better.

Day 39

AEROBIC EXERCISE

Increase your time today by 15 seconds for a total of 2 minutes and 45 seconds. You should have no trouble at all making it through the entire exercise time. At the end, walk around slowly and breathe deeply to warm down.

WEIGHT TRAINING AND STRETCHING

Today you do the Day-29 program for the pulling muscles of the upper body. Have you noticed that you feel the effects in your biceps when you do chins and rowing motions? This is due to the fact that the biceps are worked when back-pulling movements are done. After doing the back exercises, your biceps are already warmed up, so that the following exercises will have an added effect, giving you a better pump and better development.

Day 40

AEROBIC EXERCISE

Set your timer today for a full 3 minutes. Get ready, take a deep breath and exhale. Now begin the High Kicks. Keep your form under control and the pace of the exercise quick. When you have finished the 3-minute time, warm down for at least 5 minutes. Stay completely aware of all the sensations both inside and outside your body.

WEIGHT TRAINING AND STRETCHING

Repeat the Day-30 program today and really exercise your chest, shoulders, triceps and abdominal muscles deeply. Try a little music with your workouts, if you haven't already. Music adds variety and helps you develop a rhythm to your repetitions. Any kind of music is fine, just so that it pleases your partner, yourself and those around you.

Day 41

AEROBIC EXERCISE

If you have been doing a lot of walking, running or jogging in conjunction with your program, you are probably finding High Kicks easier to do. Never skip your aerobic exercises unless you are ill or overtired. In this way they will become easier for you to do. For High Kicks set your timer for 3 minutes and 15 seconds. Stretch your legs, particularly the hamstrings and calf muscles. When you are loose and relaxed, begin the exercise, gradually increasing your pace. Today try to move a little more quickly than yesterday, but be certain that your form is always correct. When you are finished, walk slowly and take your pulse using the second hand on your watch. Your pulse will slow down as you slow down, so take it right away. The rate will most likely be over 120 beats per minute. After 5 minutes of slow walking and warming down, take your pulse again. It should be under 120. If not, you are probably pushing yourself too hard and tomorrow you should listen to your body and be alert to any signs of exertion. If you are overexerting, slow your pace. Your breathing can also be an indicator of whether you are doing too much in your aerobic exercises. If you can't get your breathing back to normal or to a more normal rate after about 10 minutes of resting, you will want to take this as a warning sign and slow down your pace. Everyone has a different point at which overexertion occurs; therefore you should become increasingly aware of your body and how it speaks to you. Keep up the good work!

WEIGHT TRAINING AND STRETCHING

Repeat Day 31 today and work your legs and waistline. After you have finished today's workout, you will be halfway through your total 12-week program. You've made good progress, and you will make even more dramatic improvement in the 6 weeks ahead.

Day 42

AEROBIC EXERCISE, WEIGHT TRAINING AND STRETCHING

Today is your day of rest, so go out and enjoy yourself. Attend some sporting event, a ballet or musical show. Notice how athletes and performers move. Think about your movements during your exercise periods each day. How can you improve them?

MUTUAL-ASSISTANCE TECHNIQUE

Your attitude while working out affects not only your partner's attitude, but also the quality of the entire workout. Are you setting a good example for your partner to follow? Is he/she setting a good example for you? How can you improve your attitude and behavior?

Are you still getting sore from your workouts? Soreness means progress, but excessive soreness should be avoided. If you're very sore, rest longer between sets (30 seconds more) and do one less set of all exercises. As soon as the soreness subsides, go back to your former workout style.

BODY AWARENESS

You should have received your photos by this time. Study them very carefully. Look at all the angles and aspects of your body. What would you like to change? Make a list. Study these photos so thoroughly that you can close your eyes and easily re-create them in your mind's eye. Are there any parts of your body that would be a challenge to reshape? If so, look at these areas in the photograph, and after you have studied them well, re-create them in your mind. Keep doing this until every part is clear to you.

Stand in front of a mirror and look at yourself. Now compare what you see with the photos that you had taken on Day 35. List all of the changes that have occurred during this time. Be specific. What did you do to cause the changes? Write down your conclusions in detail.

Using a soft pencil and tracing paper, trace over the photos, outlining your body. Do all four views. After you have finished, use an eraser to make all the changes you wish. If you want to widen your shoulders and chest, and reduce your waist and hips, do this now. Place these drawings in your journal.

Date a page in your journal. Write down your feelings about the Body Awareness activities that you've done so far. Always record what comes to mind first. Don't try to figure out or intellectualize what you are writing down. Let all your feelings flow in a free and unrestricted way.

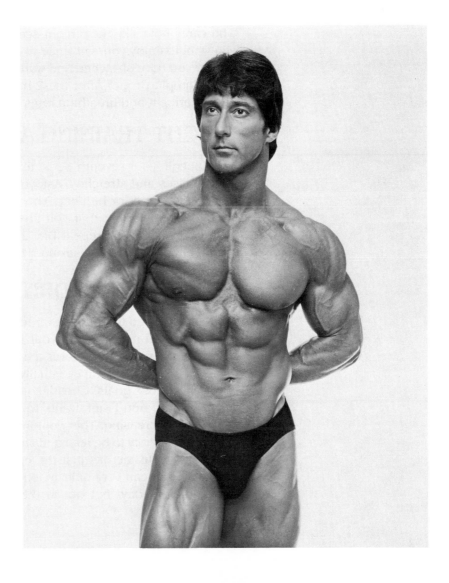

Week Seven
Day 43

AEROBIC EXERCISE

Sometimes we don't feel like exercising. Our mood might be a little low, but we feel fine physically. If this happens to you, try to think only positive thoughts. We know this is difficult, but as you will see positive thinking can bring you out of this uncertain, negative mood and elevate your spirit tremendously in a very short time. Look forward to doing your exercises. Right now, whether you are "up" or "down," think about all the positive benefits that you've already derived, and all the positive benefits you are soon to derive from your 2 minutes of aerobic work. We know of several people who like to make a game of their training. They imagine that they are in a big race or competition with a real or mythical character. If you are jumping rope, as you are today, you might visualize yourself as a kangaroo bobbing across the plains or a petite bunny hopping through a beautiful, flower-filled meadow. These images may seem silly; but no one knows what you are thinking, and if these little tricks help you to get through your jumping, then who cares how silly they might seem? It is the result that you're after, and you want to enjoy yourself while you're reaping the benefits.

After you have stretched and warmed up, set your timer for 2 minutes and begin jumping rope. After the 2-minute time period, cool down and allow your heartbeat and breathing rates to return to normal.

WEIGHT TRAINING AND STRETCHING

As you begin your seventh week, think of how you can improve your form in the exercises and stretches. Ask your partner to watch all your movements and do the same for him/her. Then study the exercise photos and descriptions to make certain that you are doing the exercises and stretches correctly. Today you will repeat Day 29 and exercise the pulling muscles and waistline. You should feel stronger today, so use a little more weight.

INTERMEDIATE DIET TIP

Whether you need to build your body by putting on muscle and very little fat or whether you need to trim your body of excess fat and keep the muscle size to a minimum, your diet is a main factor. By recording your habits and the foods you eat you will eventually be able to custom design your eating to fit either of those goals. Christine would like to keep her muscle size and fat content down, and Frank wants to keep his muscle size increasing and his fat content decreasing. This wouldn't be much of a challenge if Christine had a natural tendency to be lean and small, and Frank had the tendency to grow, but we don't. In fact it's just the opposite. Christine grows very easily and Frank can get lean very quickly. Basically we eat the same foods and at the same times of day, but not in the same amounts. Frank may even have another meal or snack during the day, while Christine cuts down the size of her meals as the day progresses. We show you here and in the menu section how easily these two modes of eating can be accommodated in the same household without any extra toil.

Building your body takes time—in fact, you'll build a body of better quality if you do take time. Weight that is gained quickly is usually more fat than muscle. Fat is easily put on; and to keep from getting into a trend of excess fat accumulation, rather than of high-quality muscle tissue building, you will be eating a higher-protein and moderate-fat diet—with less emphasis on those "quick energy" foods such as fruits and grains. When these foods are eaten in abundance, over and above what is immediately needed for instant energy, fat is deposited on your body. Your body will store more than you'll ever find use for if you let it get out of control. You will soon be able to listen to the messages your body sends you, and give it the right amount it needs for what it is going to be doing. Interpreting your record book objectively plays an important part in giving your body the correct foods, in the proper amounts, and at the right times. Sometimes you can be eating the right foods and in the correct amounts and still gain fat. Therefore you should look at the times when you are eating. Meals should be regular. Eating a huge breakfast and then not eating again all day could cause your body to "think" it will be starved on a regular basis, and that it should take precautions and store up for occasions like this. Often skipping meals can trigger this cycle: You eat a small amount early in the morning and at 11:00 A.M. it's lunchtime; you're not hungry so you just skip lunch. At 1:00 P.M. you're hungry but have to wait until dinner (or grab a candy bar, which we consider worse!). By the time dinner rolls around, you are starving, so you begin eating too quickly and thus overeat. Now it is late in the day, and you've eaten more than your body will require for energy purposes before you go to bed. Most likely you will put on excess fat from this. Your body is fearful that it will be starved again and wants to arm itself by storing up some fat to live off of in the future. The next day you get up to eat breakfast, and you're not hungry because you're still full from last evening's meal. Therefore you either have a very poor breakfast or skip it entirely. Thus the cycle begins again and repeats and repeats and repeats . . . .

Keep your meals regular and eat something at each scheduled meal. This will help keep your body metabolizing and eliminating on a regular basis. Your food will be used more efficiently. For the building diet you should eat a very substantial breakfast high in protein, and keep the amount of grain products and coffee and tea to a minimum. If you are drinking milk you should stick to 8 ounces of low-fat or whole milk, or substitute yogurt for it. Milk contains lactose (milk sugar), which could cause excess fat to be deposited on your body if it isn't used right away for energy. Don't drink too much milk, especially if you have an intolerance to digesting dairy products or if you tend to be fat. Excess milk products may also cause a buildup of mucus in the upper respiratory tract. The extra protein in your diet will help build your body and nourish and repair the tissues more quickly. Now that you are eating more protein you will notice that your muscle tone, skin, hair and nails all appear healthier. Always keep your meals high in protein. Remember that as the day progresses your meals should get lighter, because you will not be needing the same amount of energy as you do at the start of your day.

Trimming your body of excess fat doesn't require as much will power as you might assume. It is important to make an intelligent selection of foods and to choose the most effective times for eating. For trimming, start the day with a good high-protein menu, but the protein intake should be less than for someone who wants to build muscle. In the menu section we give examples to follow. Keep the amounts of food eaten at one time small, and eat slowly. Stop when your stomach is nearly full. Resting for a few minutes during the meal can keep you from overindulging. The message that you're full will arrive before you have eaten everything your eyes would like you to eat.

The general rule for trimming is to eat protein in smaller portions, fats and grains in lesser amounts and mainly in the morning, and more cleansing foods (such as low-carbohydrate vegetables and fruits with a higher fiber content, to help clean waste from your system).

Day 44

AEROBIC EXERCISE

Your aerobic work for today will begin after you have done some preliminary stretching and general warming up. When you are ready, set your timer for 2 minutes and 15 seconds. Begin jumping rope, keeping a steady rhythm for the duration of the exercise. Spend an ample amount of time afterward warming down to return your bodily functions to normal.

WEIGHT TRAINING AND STRETCHING

Do you perspire a lot when you exercise, or do you barely sweat at all? Some perspiration is beneficial because it helps remove excess toxins from your body, but you shouldn't be dripping wet. If you are sweating too much, check the temperature and humidity of your training environment and lower them if necessary. An air conditioner is often useful in the summertime, especially in high-humidity climates.

Today repeat the Day-30 program for the upper-body pushing muscles and waistline.

Day 45

AEROBIC EXERCISE

Set your timer for 2 minutes and 30 seconds, following your warm-up. Begin the Jump Rope exercise. You should be averaging about 60 jumps per minute. When you're finished, follow with a thorough warm-down period of slow walking.

WEIGHT TRAINING AND STRETCHING

Exercise your legs and waist with the Day-31 program. It is important to wear appropriate clothing so that you are not too cold or too hot during your workout. Wear clothing that is loose enough to permit a full range of movement for all your exercises.

Day 46

AEROBIC EXERCISE

After loosening and thoroughly warming up your shoulders, legs and arms set your timer for 2 minutes and 45 seconds, and begin Jump Rope. Afterward, finish off the aerobic period by walking slowly and cooling down.

WEIGHT TRAINING AND STRETCHING

Repeat the Day-29 program for the pulling muscles and abdominals. The forearm muscles are very important for a strong grip and for preventing elbow injuries. Stronger, better-developed forearms mean stronger elbows as well. One of the best exercises for the forearms is the Wrist Curl (see page 95).

Day 47

AEROBIC EXERCISE

Set your timer for 3 minutes of Jump Rope today. This exercise becomes easier the more you practice. It is one of the best conditioning exercises that we know of.

WEIGHT TRAINING AND STRETCHING

Repeat Day 30 for the pushing muscles and waistline. You should always get a good pump from this program, because most of the exercises work more than one muscle group. Are you still keeping your rest periods to a minimum, not exceeding 1½ to 2 minutes? It is much better to do your workout quickly and to get it completed rather than wasting time in the gym doing the same workout in a longer period of time.

Day 48

AEROBIC EXERCISE

Today set your timer for 3 minutes and 15 seconds after a thorough warm-up. Begin Jump Rope and after you have completed the vigorous workout, take plenty of time to warm down and return to a more relaxed state.

WEIGHT TRAINING AND STRETCHING

Today is your last workout day of Week 7. Do the leg and waist program of Day 31. We hope that you are feeling more and more accomplished and that your physical goals are becoming more real as you continue. Really work for a good pump in your calves during all of the calf exercises and stretches.

Day 49

AEROBIC EXERCISE, WEIGHT TRAINING AND STRETCHING

Today is your day of rest. Relax and do whatever you feel like doing as long as it is healthy and in your best interest. Every rest day think about how much closer you are to reaching your goal.

MUTUAL-ASSISTANCE TECHNIQUE

Praise something that your partner is doing well. How can you further improve your workouts? Do you speak positively when working out, or do you complain and/or blame others? If you speak in a positive way of your training, your attitude will improve and so will the quality of what you are doing. Always ask yourself if your attitude is right before you begin.

BODY AWARENESS

Whether or not you feel you are talented in an artistic way will not affect the outcome of today's exercise. Using a page in your journal, divide it into four equal sections. In two sections write the word *now*. In the other two sections write the word *after*. In the "now" sections draw yourself from memory in two different views. Include as much detail as you can. Next, draw yourself in the sections marked "after" in the same views but in the way you will look at the end of your 12-week program. Again be specific, but also be reasonable. Miracles, like being taller or shorter at the end of the program, can't be expected to happen! When you are finished, study each drawing and go over in your mind the changes that you will need to make to meet these expectations.

On Day 35 you listed the changes that you wanted to see by the twelfth week. Using a tape recorder, tape these changes in the present tense. For example, if one of your goals is "I will reduce my waistline," then say aloud on tape, "I have a small waistline with a flat abdomen." After dictating a change, pause for a few seconds and then state the next change on your list in the present tense. When you have completed the tape, rewind it and have it ready for use. (If you don't have access to a tape recorder, write down these goals in the present tense.)

Now, using the tape you just recorded, find a quiet place where you can sit or lie down and not be disturbed. Get comfortable and then turn on the tape. Close your eyes and visualize as vividly as you can what you are listening to. See colors; feel sensations and notice if there are any emotions involved. If you wrote your changes, read them aloud one at a time. After each one close your eyes and visualize it.

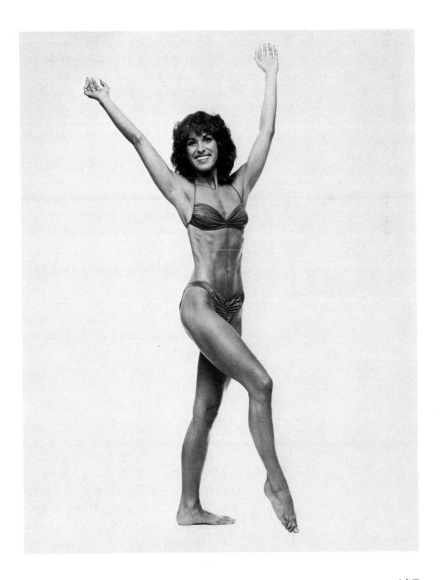

Week Eight
Day 50

AEROBIC EXERCISE

Today instead of beginning the Track Start at 2 minutes as you did in the Basic Program, you'll begin at 3 minutes and increase your time each day by 15 seconds. At the end of this week you'll be doing 4 minutes and 15 seconds of aerobic work as opposed to your previous 3 minutes and 15 seconds. This will give you added stamina and endurance.

Set the timer for 3 minutes even, after you have done a thorough warm-up of stretching the hamstrings, ankles and back. If you don't completely remember the form of this movement, reread the suggestions on Week 4 of the Basic Program. In fact, we believe that no matter how advanced you feel you are, you should become a beginner again occasionally and refresh your memory about the technique and style of the movements you work with the most.

Begin the Track Start and keep your pace quick. Don't drag your feet along the ground as you change legs. Get a good bounce and hop, so that you glide above the ground easily. You'll feel this exercise more effectively if you do it this way. Warm down completely, shaking out your legs and arms.

WEIGHT TRAINING AND STRETCHING

Repeat Day 29. Of course, by now you're using more weight, but the exercises are the same. Increase your barbell weight by 5 pounds and your dumbbell weight by 2½ pounds each over the poundages you used last week. By increasing the weight each week you will become stronger and your muscles will develop faster.

INTERMEDIATE DIET TIP

Snacks—have you been having any? If so, have they been within the guidelines of your goals? Did you have them because you were physically hungry? If not, you are eating more than your body needs and most likely you'll start seeing these snacks as extra "baggage" on your body. If you must have snacks, choose very light, low-carbohydrate vegetables or high-protein foods in small portions. If you are really hungry between meals, maybe you aren't eating enough at mealtimes. If you enjoy snacking, then make your meals smaller and distribute them evenly from morning to late afternoon. This is an excellent way to eat as long as you don't have full meals each time —which is sometimes difficult if you're trimming. You always tend to eat more than you normally would. In this case, what we suggest is that you pre-plan your meals and list all the foods you will eat that day, checking them off as you eat them. Do this for each day without adding any foods as you go. Once you have written them down, stick to it. You may end up not eating everything listed—that's okay. It's always better to feel satisfied than to feel stuffed. We often like to have some curried, broiled chicken wings prepared ahead and ready to eat cold for small, high-protein snacks. These can be made at the same time as other meat dishes and not take any extra time or energy. There are a lot of finger foods in the recipe section from which to choose. Always be sure your snacks are fresh, not processed.

Keep in mind that on your days off from exercising you may not be expending as much energy as you normally would, and therefore lighter meals would be in order. Lighter meals one day a week will give your system a chance to rest. See the recipe and menu sections for suggestions.

Day 51

AEROBIC EXERCISE

When you do your Track Start exercise today, see if you can arrange to do it with your workout partner or someone else who is interested in aerobics. Working together makes the time go faster, picks up your pace and is more fun. Before you begin, spend ample time stretching and warming up. Then set your timer for 3 minutes and 15 seconds and begin immediately. When finished, take a slow walk with your partner and discuss your training, diet and reaching your goals.

WEIGHT TRAINING AND STRETCHING

Repeat Day 30 and use 5 pounds more in each barbell exercise and 2½ pounds more in each dumbbell exercise. Don't forget to keep track of the weight used. Look through the records you've kept so far and notice that as your workouts have improved, so have your appearance and your physical condition.

Day 52

AEROBIC EXERCISE

After a warm-up, set your timer for 3 minutes and 30 seconds. Begin Track Start. Stretch way out in the movement. Spend a good amount of time walking to warm down afterward.

WEIGHT TRAINING AND STRETCHING

Repeat Day 31 and use 5 pounds more on each barbell exercise and 2½ pounds more each dumbbell exercise. Notice how your legs are getting stronger each week and how the weights are feeling lighter.

Day 53

AEROBIC EXERCISE

Begin with a slow, methodical approach to your warm-up. Use some of the warm-up exercises that you have used for your legs, back and arms in the weight-training and stretching portions of your program. When ready, set your timer for 3 minutes and 45 seconds and begin Track Start. Walk around and stretch when you are through.

WEIGHT TRAINING AND STRETCHING

Repeat Day 29 and today try to use the same weights that you used on Day 50, only do the program by resting less. See if you can knock a few minutes off the total length of time that your program generally takes. We're sure you've noticed how your waistline is shaping up.

Day 54

AEROBIC EXERCISE

When you do aerobic exercises such as Track Start you create many positive effects within your body. Your blood vessels increase in strength, elasticity and number, thereby rushing blood throughout your body with more energy-producing oxygen. Your tissues are then nourished. Your resting heart rate will decrease, and your heart becomes stronger and more efficient. Each beat pumps a greater amount of blood; therefore fewer beats are necessary. A heart that has to beat very fast to pump blood through the body is a sign of the need for conditioning. The best way to condition your heart is through aerobics. So get started today by doing some good, thorough warm-ups and then set your timer for 4 minutes and begin the Track Start. Remember your warm-down period afterward. You don't want to shock your system by stopping too suddenly. Keep moving slowly to return your heart rate and breathing to closer to normal.

WEIGHT TRAINING AND STRETCHING

Repeat Day 30 using the same poundages as earlier in the week on Day 51. This time, however, try to cut down a little on your rest periods to make your entire workout a few minutes shorter. By doing this you make greater demands on your heart, circulatory system and lungs. Your endurance will also improve. Training this way complements your aerobic work and vice versa. Always be aware of how long your workouts take.

Day 55

AEROBIC EXERCISE

As with your heart pumping more blood with less work, something similar happens with regard to your lungs. Regular aerobic work causes you to breathe more deeply for longer periods of time. Your lungs become conditioned to doing more work and can handle more oxygen with less effort. Your body receives this benefit in the form of increased energy. Most people don't even use a fraction of the full capacity of their lungs. Aerobics help increase the lungs' capacity as you breathe more deeply and exhale more completely. Your breathing is no longer shallow. Your breath is your life. We have heard it said: The fewer breaths you have to take naturally, the longer your life. This is a great incentive for doing aerobics on a regular basis!

After warm-up, set your timer for 4 minutes and 15 seconds, and begin Track Start. After finishing, breathe deeply and concentrate on filling your lungs just as you would fill a glass with water. Start filling the bottom, then the middle and then the top. When you exhale, empty first the top of your lungs, then the middle and last all the way completely to the bottom. Get in the habit of breathing deeply like this at least several times a day. Begin with a few breaths and gradually increase as you feel you are able to.

WEIGHT TRAINING AND STRETCHING

Repeat Day 31 and use the same weights for your exercises as you did on Day 52, but rest a little less between sets. Your breathing may not have returned quite to normal as you begin your next set, but by cultivating the "breathless state" in this manner you will naturally get your breath back and more quickly, the longer you practice this method. The less time you need to recover between sets, the better shape you are in.

Day 56

AEROBIC EXERCISE, WEIGHT TRAINING AND STRETCHING

Today is your rest day, and it marks the completion of your Intermediate Program. Congratulations! You are a lot closer to achieving your goal, which is now only 4 weeks away. Get a good rest. Don't be afraid to indulge in other forms of recreational exercise; just don't wear yourself out, because tomorrow you go on to the Advanced Program, which makes progressively more strenuous demands on your body.

MUTUAL-ASSISTANCE TECHNIQUE

Today eat at least one meal with your partner. Write down everything you eat and drink for all meals as usual. How many calories, carbohydrates, proteins and fats did you consume today? How can you improve your food selections and eating habits? How can you help your partner improve his/her diet? Get to know your partner even better today. Tell him/her exactly how you want to improve your diet and if he/she has any suggestions that could be helpful to you. While eating your nutritiously prepared meal together keep in mind the deliciousness of the food and that with each mouthful you are getting in better and better shape and closer and closer to your goal.

INTERMEDIATE PROGRAM	First Level			Middle Level			Top Level		
Day-29 Exercises	Weight Used	Sets	Reps	Weight Used	Sets	Reps	Weight Used	Sets	Reps
Dumbbell Shrug									
Downward Neck Stretch									
Wide-Grip Chins or Letdowns									
Sideways Swing									
Barbell Row									
One-Arm Lat Stretch									
Barbell Curl									
Arms Backward Stretch with Pronation									
Alternate Dumbbell Curl									
Push-ups, Fingers Back Stretch									
Wrist Curl									
Wall Lean (for forearms)									
Reverse Curl									
Fist Curl, Wrist Down									
Incline Knee-in									

BODY AWARENESS

Using your tape recorder (or writing a list), record 10 positive aspects of yourself that have emerged as a result of the last 8 weeks of training and diet. After each idea, pause for 30 seconds.

Find a quiet place to lie down or sit, where you are comfortable and won't be disturbed. With your eyes closed, replay the tape recording you just made. Clearly visualize everything you're listening to. During the 30-second pause, bring your visualizations into more focused detail.

Replay this recording again and, as you listen, sketch the changes you have mentioned. Do them very quickly, focusing only on the specifics. (If you wrote the ideas, spend about 1 minute on each sketch and then move to the next one.)

Date a new page in your journal in the Body Awareness section, and write down all the ideas and feelings, as they come to you, about the exercises you have done thus far.

INTERMEDIATE PROGRAM	First Level			Middle Level			Top Level		
Day-30 Exercises	Weight Used	Sets	Reps	Weight Used	Sets	Reps	Weight Used	Sets	Reps
Push-ups (warm-up)									
Bench Press									
Doorway Stretch									
Dumbbell Fly									
Incline Stretch Between Chairs									
Dumbbell Press									
One-Arm Shoulder Stretch									
Dumbbell Side Raise									
Doorway Isometric Lateral Stretch									
Dumbbell Rear Raise									
Doorway Isometric Front Stretch									
Close-Grip Bench Press									
Reverse Dip Between Chairs									
Two-Arm Dumbbell Extension									
Arms-Backward Stretch									
Incline Knee-in									
Bent-Leg Partial Sit-up									

INTERMEDIATE PROGRAM	First Level			Middle Level			Top Level		
Day-31 Exercises	Weight Used	Sets	Reps	Weight Used	Sets	Reps	Weight Used	Sets	Reps
One-Leg Top Extension (warm-up)									
Half Squat									
Lunge with Back Foot on Bench									
Hack Squat									
Forward Stretch									
Stiff-Legged Deadlift									
One-Leg-up Stretch									
Donkey Calf Raise									
Two-Leg Calf Stretch									
One-Leg Calf Raise									
Wall Lean (for calves)									
Incline Knee-In									
Bent-Leg Partial Sit-up									
Seated Twist									

ADVANCED PROGRAM

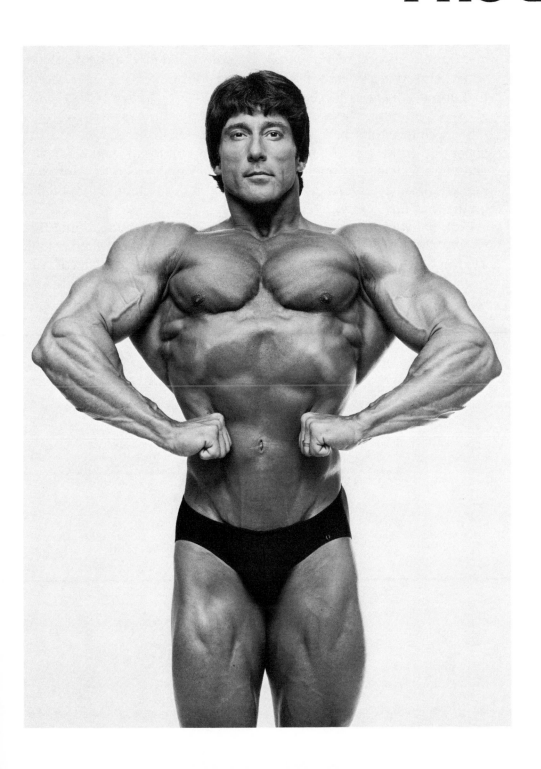

Introduction

This is the final stage of your program. You'll still be working the whole body in 3 days, as in the Intermediate Program (first day—back, biceps, forearms, waist; second day—chest, shoulders, triceps, waist; and third day—legs and waist). But you will be doing more exercises and sets per body part. You will need additional equipment to follow the program. The extra equipment includes: a lat pulldown machine, a leg extension and leg curl machine, and a standing calf machine. You'll also need to have weights to make a barbell of up to 230 pounds and dumbbells up to 65 pounds each. (More weight may be needed if you're stronger and less if you aren't as strong.) Don't use weights that are too heavy or too light for you. If you don't have access to the above equipment, choose a gym that has these things along with the other weight equipment you have used so far. If necessary you can substitute Wide Grip Chins or Letdowns for Pulldowns; Leg Extension and Leg Curl can be done by using resistance supplied by your partner; and Donkey Calf Raise can be substituted for Standing Calf Raise on the machine.

In the advanced section you will increase the amount of time that you hold all your stretches and cut your rest periods between sets to 1½ minutes from the previous 2 minutes. Eventually you will cut your rests to 1 minute. Plan to reach your goal at the end of the next 4 weeks!!

Here is your Day-57 program. Continue at the same level you've been doing in the Intermediate Program (First, Middle or Top level). This program will be done on Days 60, 64, 67, 71, 74, 78 and 81.

EXERCISE	Page	First Level	Middle Level	Top Level
Hyperextension	158	1 set, 10 reps	2 sets, 15 reps	3 sets, 20 reps
Forward Stretch	159	10 seconds	2 sets, 15 sec	3 sets, 20 sec
Top Deadlift and Shrug	160	1 set, 10 reps	2 sets, 8 reps	3 sets, 12 reps
Downward Neck Stretch	161	10 seconds	2 sets, 15 sec	3 sets, 20 sec
Barbell Row	162	1 set, 10 reps	2 sets, 8 reps	3 sets, 12 reps
One-Arm Lat Stretch—High	163	10 seconds	2 sets, 15 sec	3 sets, 20 sec
Front or Behind-Neck Pulldown	164	1 set, 10 reps	2 sets, 8 reps	3 sets, 12 reps
Sideways Swing	166	1 set, 10 reps	2 sets, 8 reps	3 sets, 12 reps
One-Arm Dumbbell Row	167	1 set, 10 reps	2 sets, 8 reps	3 sets, 12 reps
One-Arm Lat Stretch—Low	168	10 seconds	2 sets, 15 sec	3 sets, 20 sec
Alternate Dumbbell Curl	169	1 set, 10 reps	2 sets, 8 reps	3 sets, 12 reps
Push-ups, Fingers Back Stretch	170	10 seconds	2 sets, 15 sec	3 sets, 20 sec
Dumbbell Incline Curl	171	1 set, 10 reps	2 sets, 8 reps	3 sets, 12 reps
Arms-Backward Stretch with Pronation	172	10 seconds	2 sets, 15 sec	3 sets, 20 sec
Dumbbell Concentration Curl	173	1 set, 10 reps	2 sets, 8 reps	3 sets, 12 reps
Doorknob Isometric Curl	174	10 seconds	2 sets, 15 sec	3 sets, 20 sec
Reverse Curl	175	1 set, 10 reps	2 sets, 8 reps	3 sets, 12 reps
Fist Curl, Wrist Down	175	10 seconds	2 sets, 15 sec	3 sets, 20 sec
Wrist Curl	176	1 set, 10 reps	2 sets, 12 reps	3 sets, 15 reps
Wall Lean	176	10 seconds	2 sets, 15 sec	3 sets, 20 sec
Incline Knee-in	177	1 set, 25 reps	2 sets, 30 reps	3 sets, 35 reps
Bent-Leg Partial Sit-up	178	1 set, 25 reps	2 sets, 30 reps	3 sets, 35 reps

HYPEREXTENSION

First level: 1 set, 10 reps
Middle level: 2 sets, 15 reps
Top level: 3 sets, 20 reps

This is a new exercise in your Advanced Program. It is a fabulous movement for strengthening your lower back (spinal erector muscles). You will feel the stimulation from the upper part of your buttocks to the central part of your back. Lie face down across a high table—like the leg extension—leg curl table—with your knees just barely off the table and your upper body totally off the table on the other side. Have your partner hold your feet. Place your arms across your chest or behind your neck and inhale as you slowly lower your head toward the floor. Exhale as you slowly lift your upper body so that it is just slightly above parallel to the table. Pause momentarily and repeat.

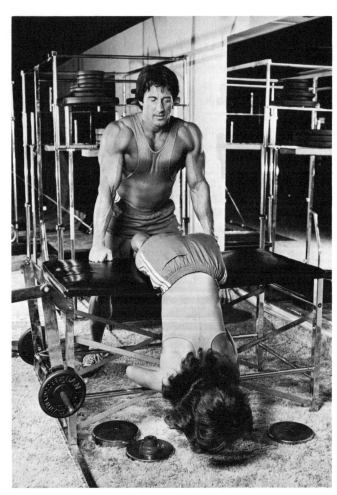

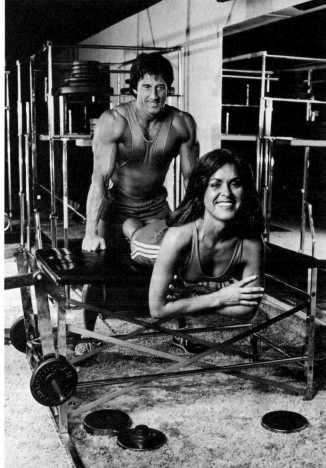

FORWARD STRETCH

First level: 1 set, 10 sec
Middle level: 2 sets, 15 sec
Top level: 3 sets, 20 sec

Do this exercise in the same manner as in the Basic Program. You should find it easier to reach a little farther down as you continue to do this stretch through the Advanced Program. Feel your hamstrings and lower back relaxing and stretching as you hold for the designated time.

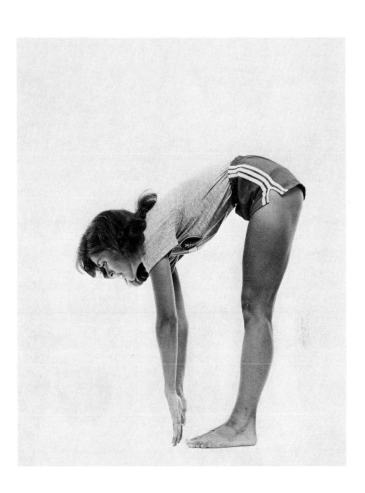

TOP DEADLIFT AND SHRUG

First level: 1 set, 10 reps
Middle level: 2 sets, 8 reps
Top level: 3 sets, 12 reps

This is a two-part movement that is new to your program. It works the middle of the lower back all the way up to the base of the neck (the trapezius at the top and the spinal erectors the full length of the spine). This is an excellent exercise for filling in the hollow of the upper back area. Stand holding the barbell in front of you and grasping it to each side of your thighs with an overhand grip. Lean forward so that the bar touches your legs just above the kneecap. Exhale as you stand up straight and then shrug your shoulders upward and slowly release the shrug. Return the bar to the above-the-knees position and repeat.

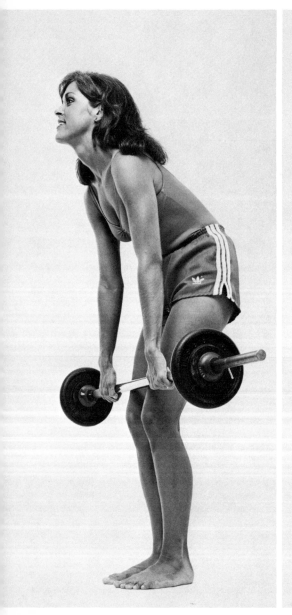
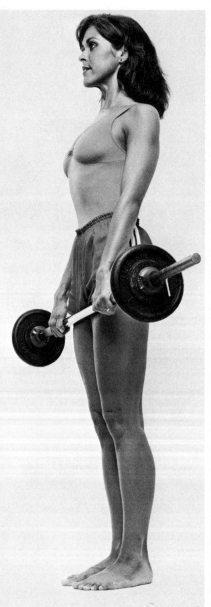
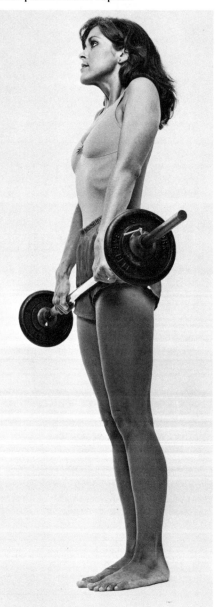

DOWNWARD NECK STRETCH

First level: 1 set, 10 sec
Middle level: 2 sets, 15 sec
Top level: 3 sets, 20 sec

This exercise really stimulates the back of your neck and the upper part of the trapezius. Continue to do it as you have been and visualize this area of the body as you hold for the designated time. This stretch is very effective when done immediately after Top Deadlift and Shrug.

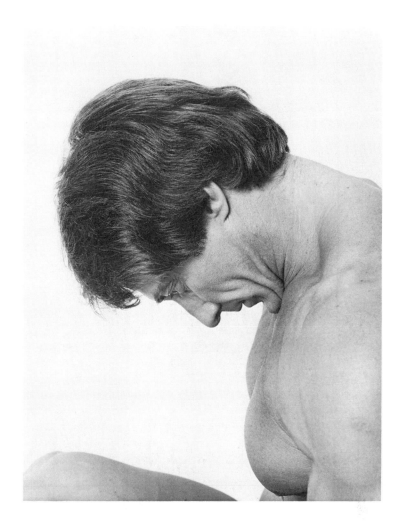

BARBELL ROW

First level: 1 set, 10 reps
Middle level: 2 sets, 8 reps
Top level: 3 sets, 12 reps

You have been doing these for over 8 weeks and by now should be developing a really good "groove" for the movement of this exercise. Be sure your knees are bent and be careful not to hit them as you raise and lower the barbell. Stretching out by rounding your back, when the barbell is at its lowest point (the weight should be lowered slowly), is the key to creating a V-shape to your back, because it develops the lower lats as well as the central portion of the latissimus dorsi muscles.

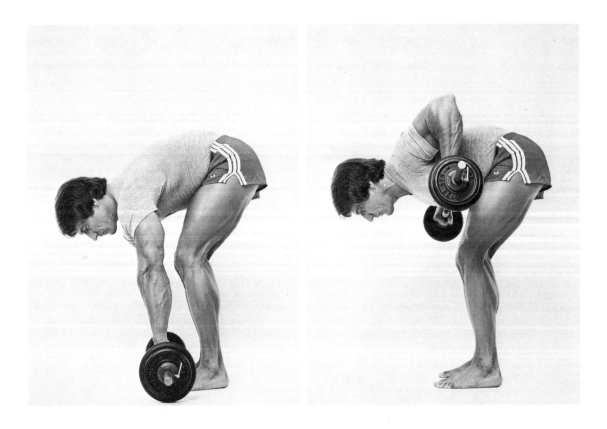

162

ONE-ARM LAT STRETCH—HIGH

First level: 1 set, 10 sec
Middle level: 2 sets, 15 sec
Top level: 3 sets, 20 sec

This exercise comes right after Barbell Row. Do it in the same way as One-Arm Lat Stretch but grip the vertical bar slightly above your head and pull downward for the designated amount of time. You'll really feel this in the V-shaped back muscles.

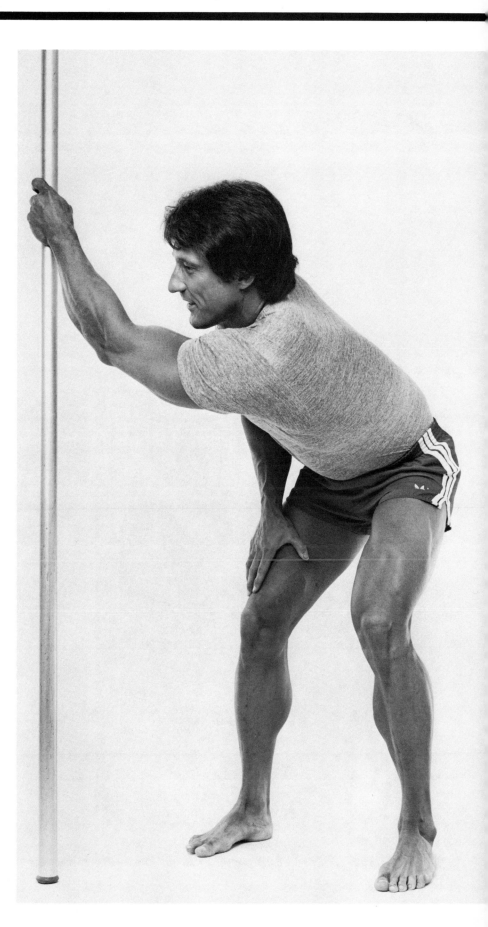

FRONT PULLDOWN

First level: 1 set, 10 reps
Middle level: 2 sets, 8 reps
Top level: 3 sets, 12 reps

This exercise works the upper back, especially the lats and serratus. Feel the area from your armpits down to the top of your rib cage expanding with each rep.

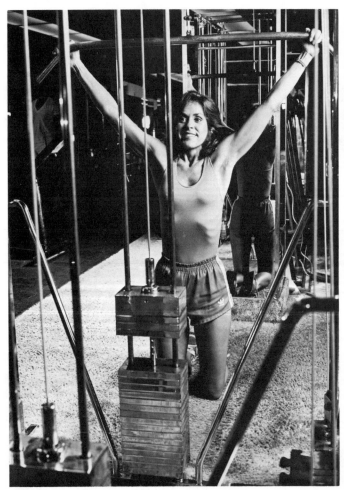
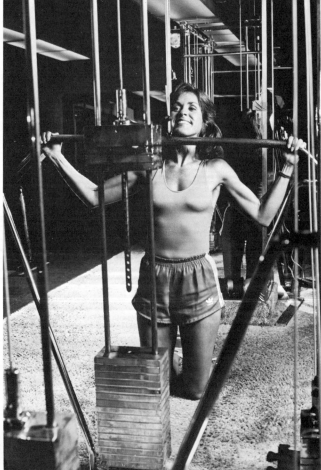

BEHIND-NECK PULLDOWN

First level: 1 set, 10 reps
Middle level: 2 sets, 8 reps
Top level: 3 sets, 12 reps

This exercise is a variation of the Front Pulldown and reaches the muscles of your upper back: lats, trapezius, teres major and minor, infraspinatus, and rear deltoids. Feel these muscles expanding as you do this exercise. Grasp the pull-down bar with a thumbless grip slightly wider than shoulder width. Inhale and pull down to the top of your chest for Front Pulldown and to the upper part of the back of your neck for Behind-Neck Pulldown. Exhale as you slowly let the lat bar return to the finish position and stretch out at this top position of the exercise.

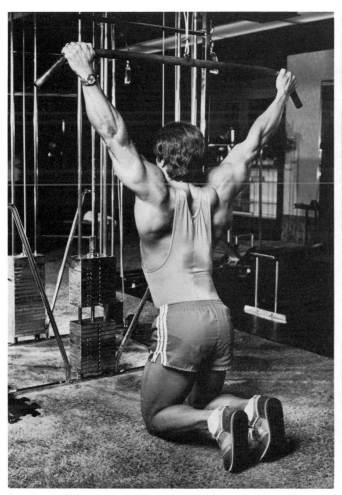
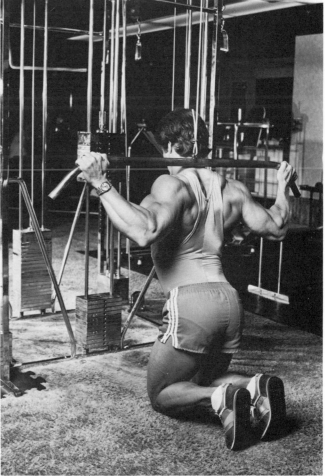

165

SIDEWAYS SWING

First level: 1 set, 10 reps
Middle level: 2 sets, 8 reps
Top level: 3 sets, 12 reps

This exercise immediately follows the Front Pulldown or Behind-Neck Pulldown. Remember that one repetition counts as you swing to both sides. Swing in both directions and get a great stretch to your lats.

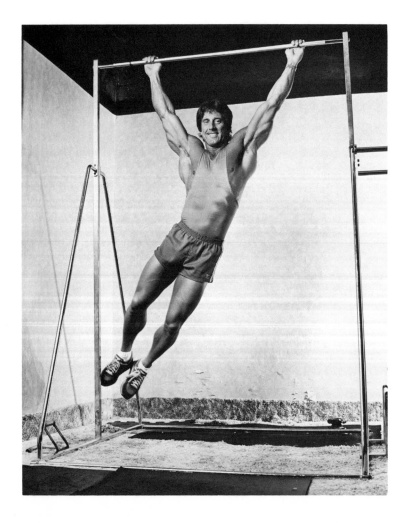

ONE-ARM DUMBBELL ROW

First level: 1 set, 10 reps
Middle level: 2 sets, 8 reps
Top level: 3 sets, 12 reps

This is a new exercise and is probably one of the most effective ways to develop the outer lats. Place your knee on a flat bench, lean forward and rest your hand on the same side of the bench (left knee and left hand rest on the right edge of the bench and vice versa). Your opposite foot will be on the floor resting on your toes, with the knee of that leg just slightly bent. The hand of that same side is extended fully down and holds a dumbbell. Bring the dumbbell up to your chest, keeping your elbow slightly in to your side. Slowly lower the dumbbell to the fully extended position. Repeat the movement. Do this same movement on the other side by switching your position. It is important to use a bench that is high enough to allow a full stretch as you lower the dumbbell to its very lowest position (almost touching the floor). This is what fully develops your lats.

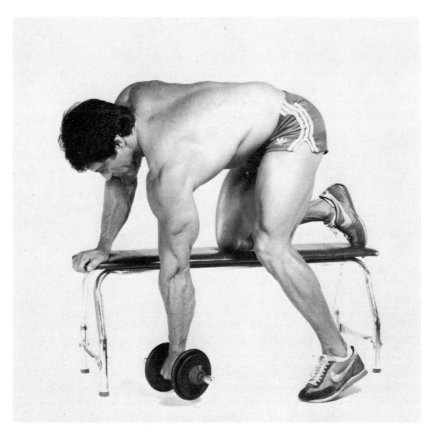

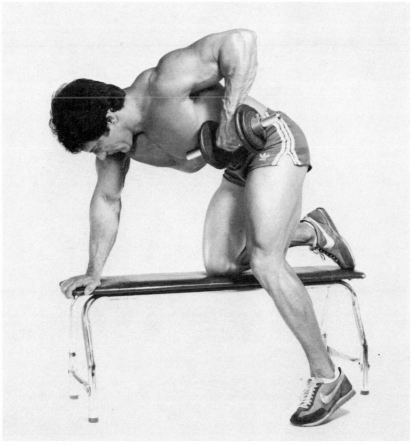

ONE-ARM LAT STRETCH—LOW

First level: 1 set, 10 sec
Middle level: 2 sets, 15 sec
Top level: 3 sets, 20 sec

Do this exercise as before, but grip the bar about 1 foot from the floor and pull upward. You'll feel the stretching effect from the lower lat and the sides of your waist. Hold the stretch for the designated time.

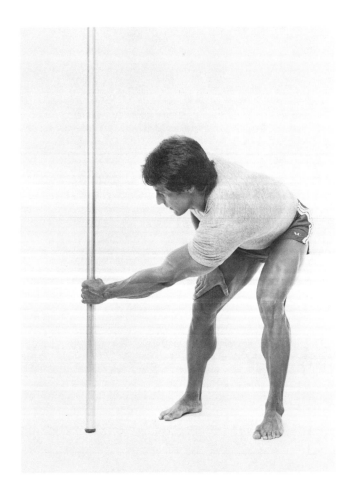

ALTERNATE DUMBBELL CURL

First level: 1 set, 10 reps
Middle level: 2 sets, 8 reps
Top level: 3 sets, 12 reps

You'll continue this exercise from the Intermediate Program as you've been doing it. This tones the frontal shoulders as well as the outer biceps. Work for a smooth rhythm in this movement.

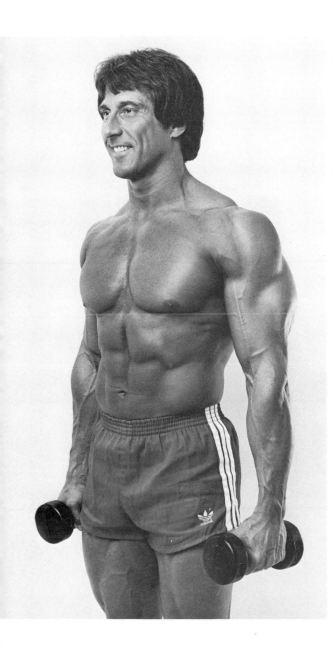
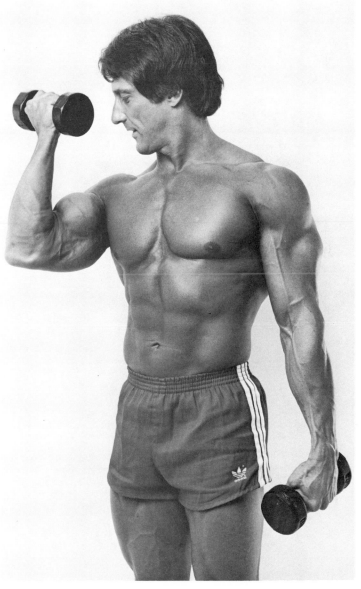

169

PUSH-UPS, FINGERS BACK STRETCH

First level: 1 set, 10 sec
Middle level: 2 sets, 15 sec
Top level: 3 sets, 20 sec

You've been doing this exercise. You should really be noticing how much stronger your grip and forearms are becoming from this stretch. The more you position your hands forward, the more difficult this stretch becomes.

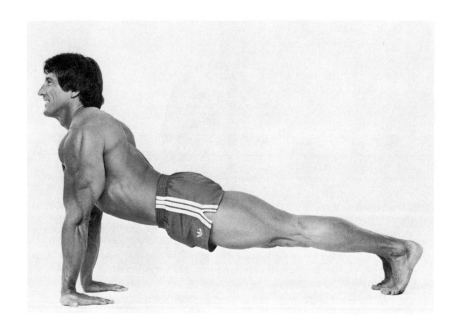

170

DUMBBELL INCLINE CURL

First level: 1 set, 10 reps
Middle level: 2 sets, 8 reps
Top level: 3 sets, 12 reps

This exercise is new to your program. It works the upper biceps more as the angle of the incline decreases. It affects the frontal deltoid and works the outer biceps when your elbows are held in close to your body. Sit back on an incline bench (about a 45-degree angle), with your arms down to each side, holding dumbbells which are turned outward. Inhale and curl the weights upward, keeping your wrist straight and your elbows close to your body. Tense your biceps at the top of the movement and then exhale as you slowly lower the dumbbell down to the starting position. You'll feel an expansive sensation in your upper, outer biceps.

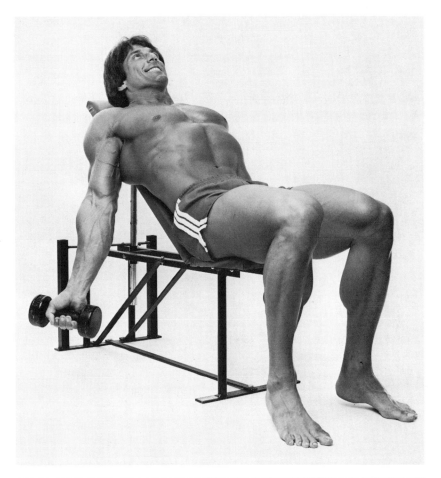

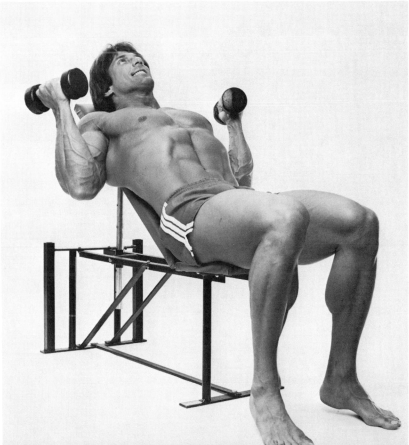

ARMS-BACKWARD STRETCH WITH PRONATION

First level: 1 set, 10 sec
Middle level: 2 sets, 15 sec
Top level: 3 sets, 20 sec

This stretch immediately follows Dumbbell Incline Curl. Do it as you've been doing it before, but this time try for a bigger stretch than ever before. Resting as little as possible, go to Dumbbell Concentration Curl.

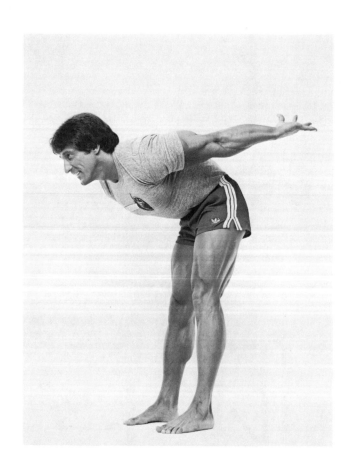

DUMBBELL CONCENTRATION CURL

First level: 1 set, 10 reps
Middle level: 2 sets, 8 reps
Top level: 3 sets, 12 reps

This exercise is best for developing height or a "peak" to your biceps. Bend at the waist with one hand on your knee and grasp a dumbbell with the other hand. Keep your wrists straight; inhale as you curl the dumbbell up until it barely touches your chin. Tense your biceps in this position. Exhale as you lower the weight to the starting position. Be sure not to move your elbow inward, toward your body, when curling up. You'll feel the stimulation in your biceps with each rep.

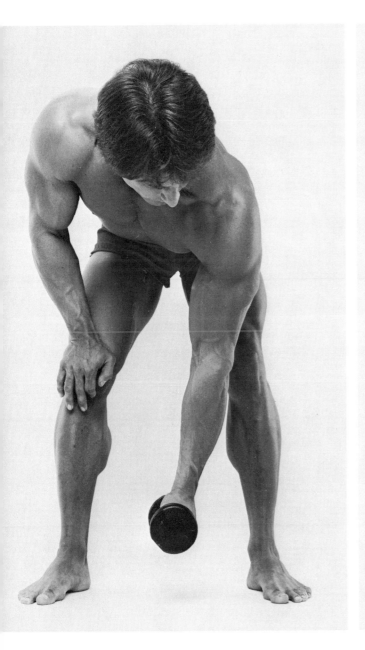
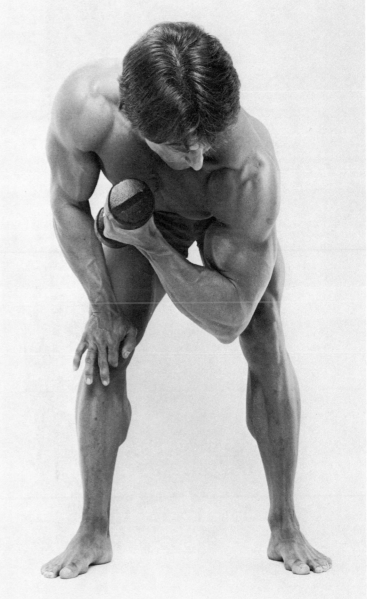

DOORKNOB ISOMETRIC CURL

First level: 1 set, 10 sec
Middle level: 2 sets, 15 sec
Top level: 3 sets, 20 sec

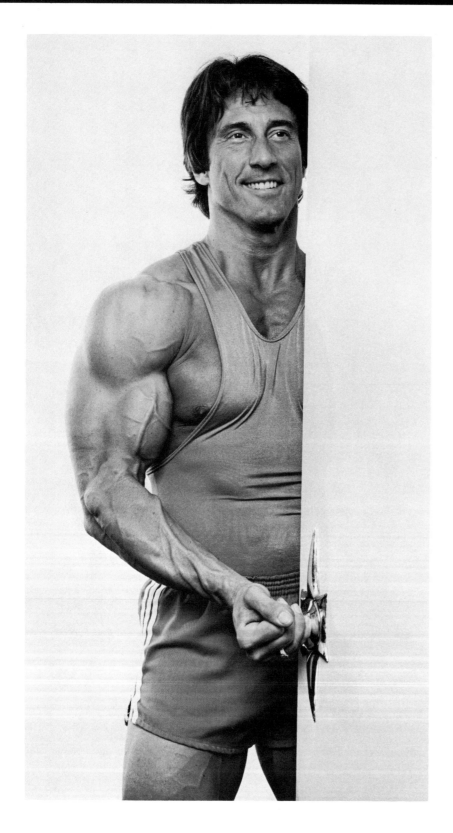

This movement will build strength and develop the lower biceps when done immediately after a curling exercise with weights. Grasp a doorknob on each side with an underhand grip and pull upward with your elbows bent. As you hold the contraction, feel your biceps getting stronger.

REVERSE CURL

First level: 1 set, 10 reps
Middle level: 2 sets, 8 reps
Top level: 3 sets, 12 reps

FIST CURL, WRIST DOWN

First level: 1 set, 10 sec
Middle level: 2 sets, 15 sec
Top level: 3 sets, 20 sec

Continue to do these two exercises—the second is the stretching movement—immediately afterward, as before. Concentrate on squeezing as hard as you can on each repetition for a maximum stimulation in your forearms. Notice how strong your wrists are getting?

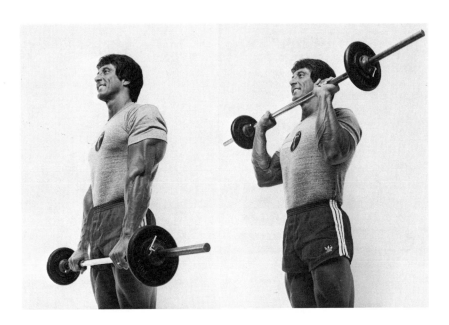

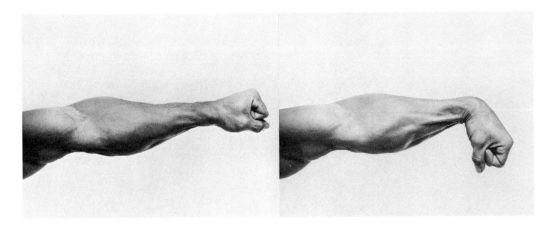

175

WRIST CURL

First level: 1 set, 10 reps
Middle level: 2 sets, 8 reps
Top level: 3 sets, 12 reps

WALL LEAN

First level: 1 set, 10 sec
Middle level: 2 sets, 15 sec
Top level: 3 sets, 20 sec

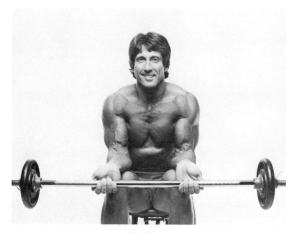

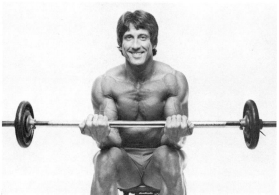

For your forearm development and grip you will be doing Wrist Curl immediately followed by Wall Lean. For Wrist Curl you'll be doing higher repetitions than in the Intermediate Program because you are stronger now. Do this exercise and the Wall Lean as before and focus in on your forearm muscles working as you do each exercise and stretch.

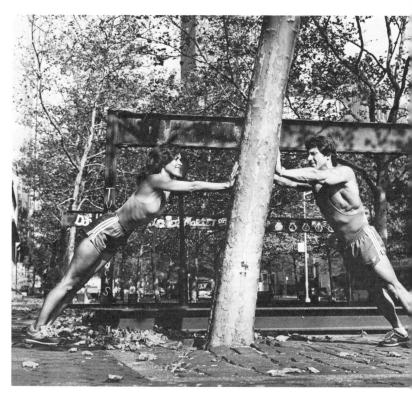

You've been working your waist for 6 days a week since you began the Intermediate Program and you should notice quite a difference in how your waistline looks. Daily work keeps the waistline trim.

INCLINE KNEE-IN

First level: 1 set, 20 reps
Middle level: 2 sets, 25 reps
Top level: 3 sets, 30 reps

Do this exercise as you have before, but you'll add more repetitions. Concentrate on the lower abdominals as you do each rep.

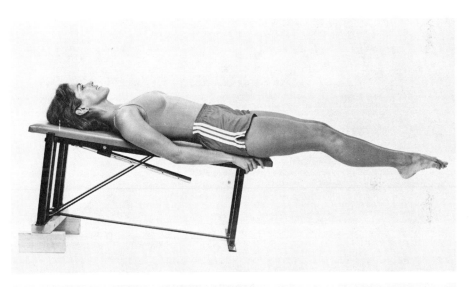

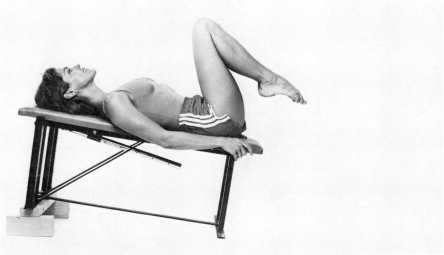

177

BENT-LEG PARTIAL SIT-UP

First level: 1 set, 20 reps
Middle level: 2 sets, 25 reps
Top level: 3 sets, 30 reps

These are also done as you've been doing them but with higher reps because your abdominals are stronger now. Feel the pulling sensation in the upper abdominals. If you raise up slightly sideways in this exercise, you'll work the sides of your waist too (intercostals and obliques).

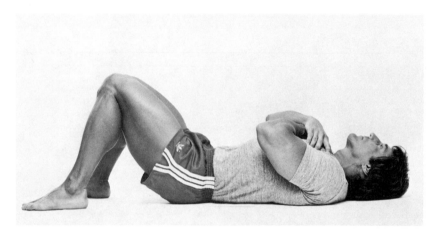

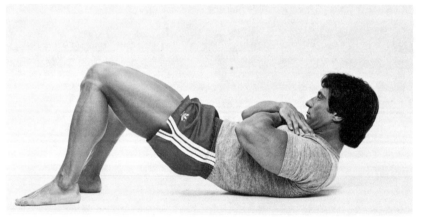

Here is your Day-58 program. It is also done on Days 61, 65, 68, 72, 75, 79 and 82.

EXERCISE	Page	First Level	Middle Level	Top Level
Push-ups (warm-up)	180	1 set, 15 reps	1 set, 15 reps	1 set, 15 reps
Bench Press	181	1 set, 10 reps	2 sets, 8 reps	3 sets, 12 reps
Doorway Stretch	182	10 seconds	2 sets, 15 sec	3 sets, 20 sec
Incline Dumbbell Press	183	1 set, 10 reps	2 sets, 8 reps	3 sets, 12 reps
Incline Stretch Between Chairs	184	10 seconds	2 sets, 15 sec	3 sets, 20 sec
Decline Dumbbell Fly	185	1 set, 10 reps	2 sets, 8 reps	3 sets, 12 reps
Pectoral Squeeze	186	10 seconds	2 sets, 15 sec	3 sets, 20 sec
Dumbbell Pullover	187	1 set, 10 reps	2 sets, 8 reps	3 sets, 12 reps
One-Arm Dumbbell Row	187	1 set, 10 reps	2 sets, 8 reps	3 sets, 12 reps
Dip Stretch Between Chairs	188	10 seconds	2 sets, 15 sec	3 sets, 20 sec
Dumbbell Press	189	1 set, 10 reps	2 sets, 8 reps	3 sets, 12 reps
One-Arm Shoulder Stretch	190	10 seconds	2 sets, 15 sec	3 sets, 20 sec
Barbell Front Raise	191	1 set, 10 reps	2 sets, 8 reps	3 sets, 12 reps
Doorknob Isometric Front Raise	192	10 seconds	2 sets, 15 sec	3 sets, 20 sec
Dumbbell Side Raise	193	1 set, 10 reps	2 sets, 8 reps	3 sets, 12 reps
Doorway Isometric Lateral Stretch	194	10 seconds	2 sets, 15 sec	3 sets, 20 sec
Dumbbell Rear Raise	195	1 set, 10 reps	2 sets, 8 reps	3 sets, 12 reps
Doorway Isometric Front Stretch	195	10 seconds	2 sets, 15 sec	3 sets, 20 sec
Close-Grip Bench Press	196	1 set, 10 reps	2 sets, 8 reps	3 sets, 12 reps
Reverse Dip Stretch Between Chairs	197	10 seconds	2 sets, 15 sec	3 sets, 20 sec
One-Arm Dumbbell Extension	198	1 set, 10 reps	2 sets, 8 reps	3 sets, 12 reps
Overhead Stretch	199	10 seconds	2 sets, 15 sec	3 sets, 20 sec
Dumbbell Kickback	200	1 set, 10 reps	2 sets, 8 reps	3 sets, 12 reps
Arms-Backward Stretch	201	10 seconds	2 sets, 15 sec	3 sets, 20 sec
Hanging Knee-up	202	1 set, 15 reps	2 sets, 20 reps	3 sets, 25 reps
Seated Twist	203	1 set, 25 reps	2 sets, 30 reps	3 sets, 35 reps

PUSH-UPS

All levels: 1 set, 10 reps

Do only one set of Push-ups of 15 reps
because it is a warm-up for Bench Press.

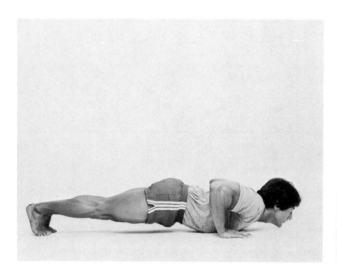
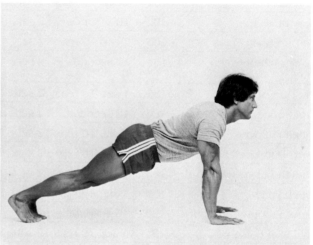
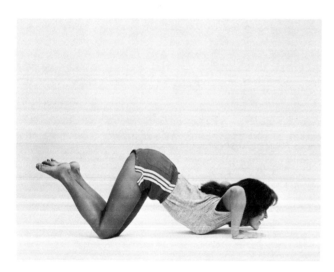
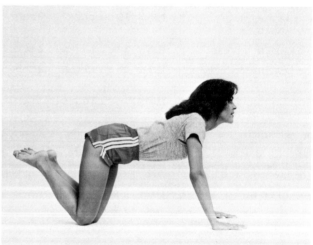

BENCH PRESS

First level: 1 set, 10 reps
Middle level: 2 sets, 8 reps
Top level: 3 sets, 12 reps

By now you should have great control over the barbell as you raise and lower it, feeling stimulation and firmness after you do each set.

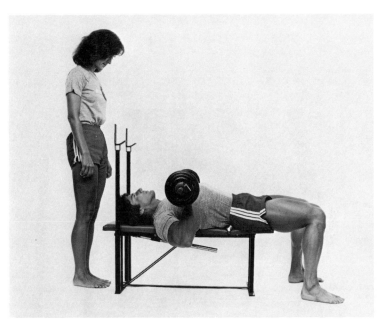

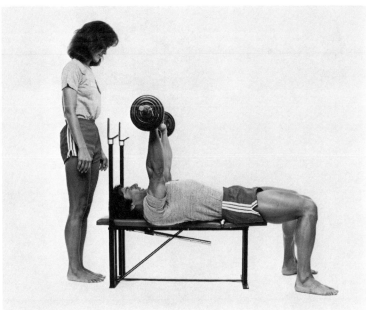

181

DOORWAY STRETCH

First level: 1 set, 10 reps
Middle level: 2 sets, 8 reps
Top level: 3 sets, 12 reps

Really get a full, deep stretch while doing this so that you can feel the increased blood circulation in your shoulder and chest areas. These first 3 exercises/ stretches bring a lot of fresh blood supply into your pushing muscles when done one after the other.

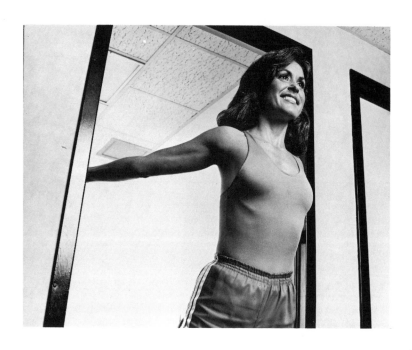

INCLINE DUMBBELL PRESS

First level: 1 set, 10 reps
Middle level: 2 sets, 8 reps
Top level: 3 sets, 12 reps

This is a new exercise for your Advanced Program. It is the most direct exercise for developing the upper part of the chest. For women this is good for preventing sagging breasts and for developing an outstanding cleavage. For both men and women this exercise will fill in the area around the clavicles. Lie on a 45-degree incline bench with dumbbells held overhead. Inhale and slowly lower the weights as far as they will go, turning your wrists outward as you do. Get a good stretch in this low position and exhale as you push the dumbbells up to the starting position.

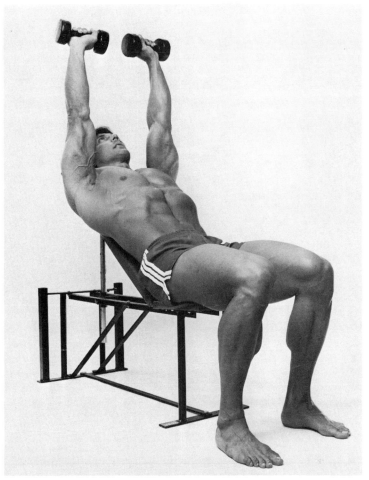

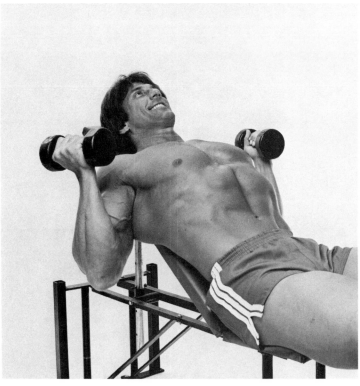

INCLINE STRETCH BETWEEN CHAIRS

First level: 1 set, 10 sec
Middle level: 2 sets, 15 sec
Top level: 3 sets, 20 sec

Do this exercise immediately after Incline Dumbbell Press. Do it as you have before, concentrating on a deep, full stretch in your chest and shoulders.

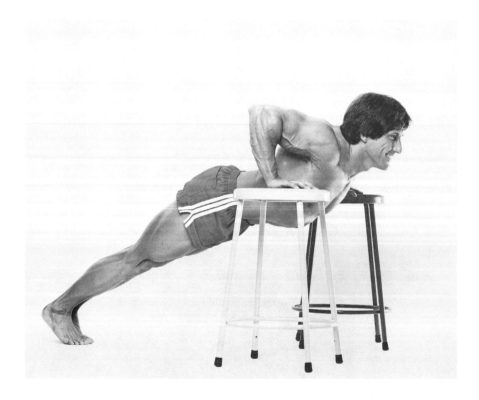

DECLINE DUMBBELL FLY

First level: 1 set, 10 reps
Middle level: 2 sets, 8 reps
Top level: 3 sets, 12 reps

This exercise is done the same way as Dumbbell Fly except that a calf block is inserted under one end of your bench to make a low decline, with your head downhill. This exercise works the lower, outer pectorals a little more directly than Dumbbell Fly, which works mainly the outer pectorals. Be sure to get a good stretch as you lower the dumbbells as far as they will go.

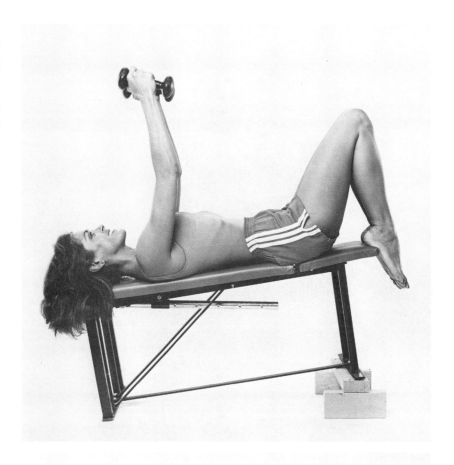

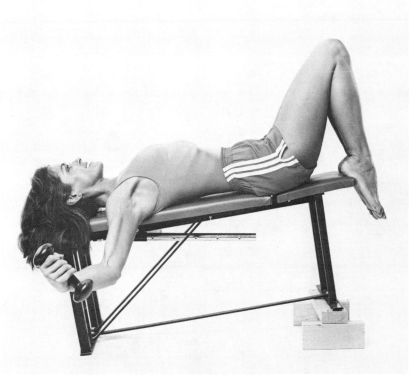

PECTORAL SQUEEZE

First level: 1 set, 10 sec
Middle level: 2 sets, 15 sec
Top level: 3 sets, 20 sec

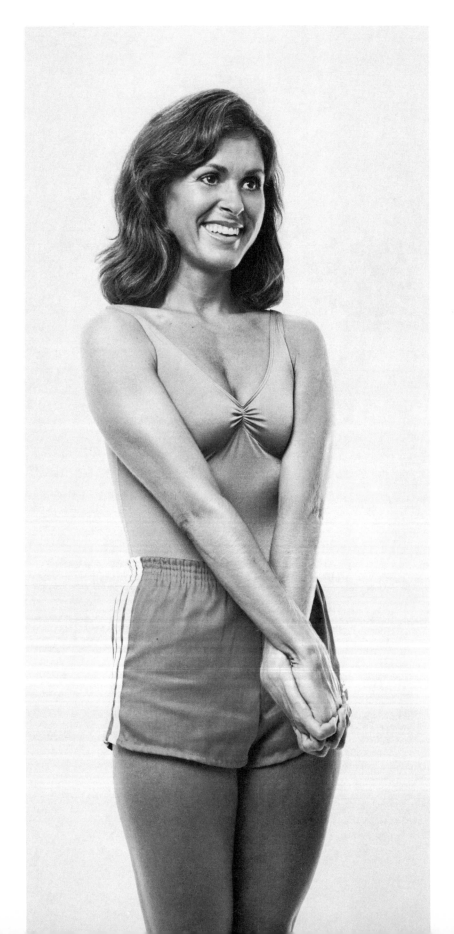

This new stretch which has been added to your program should be done immediately after Decline Dumbbell Fly. The movement contracts the inner pectoral muscles and is very beneficial for developing a cleavage. Twist each wrist inward and interlock the fingers of both hands. Squeeze your chest muscles and then relax. Feel the stimulation in the inner pectorals.

DUMBBELL PULLOVER

First level: 1 set, 10 reps
Middle level: 2 sets, 8 reps
Top level: 3 sets, 12 reps

ONE-ARM DUMBBELL ROW

First level: 1 set, 10 reps
Middle level: 2 sets, 8 reps
Top level: 3 sets, 12 reps

This is an exercise that you did in the Basic Program. Do it in the same manner as before, but use a bench that is 2 inches higher. This will allow you to stretch out more as you lower the dumbbell, and will further develop the rib cage and serratus. Your triceps also benefit from this exercise. Do the One-Arm Dumbbell Row as before.

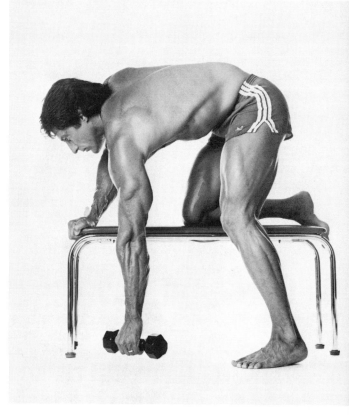

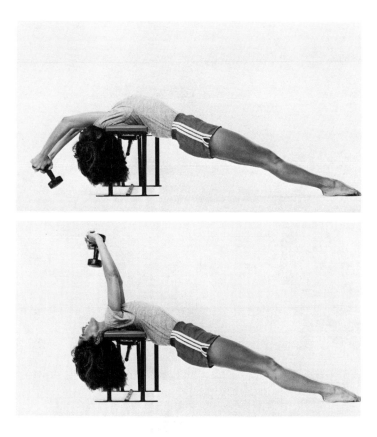

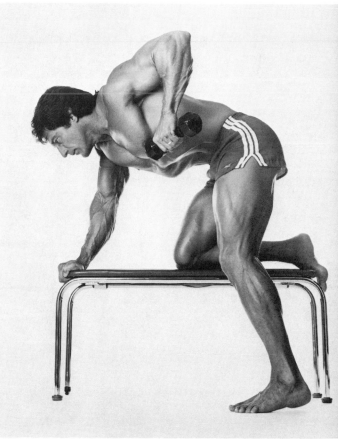

DIP STRETCH BETWEEN CHAIRS

First level: 1 set, 10 sec
Middle level: 2 sets, 15 sec
Top level: 3 sets, 20 sec

This is a new stretch for the chest and shoulders. Place two chairs facing back to back, at a distance as wide apart as your shoulders. If the chairs tend to slip, brace them with weights. Grab the back of each chair and lift your feet off the ground. Slowly lower yourself to stretch deeply below the tops of the chairs. Hold this stretch. (This exercise can also be done with two stools, as pictured.)

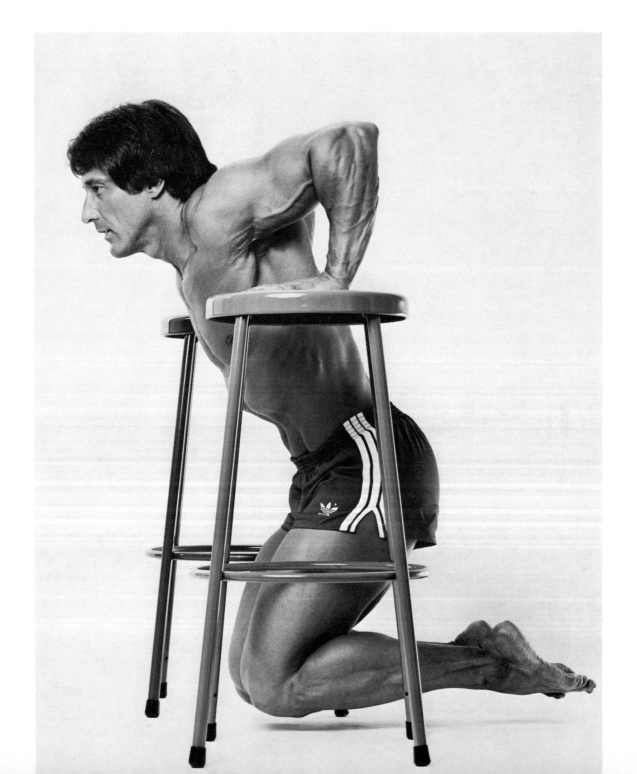

DUMBBELL PRESS

First level: 1 set, 10 reps
Middle level: 2 sets, 8 reps
Top level: 3 sets, 12 reps

Continue this exercise as before, only now try slowing down the movement a little, especially when you lower the weights. Do each rep to feel stimulation in the front and side deltoids as well as in the extreme upper portion of your chest. This exercise will give you added shoulder width and strength.

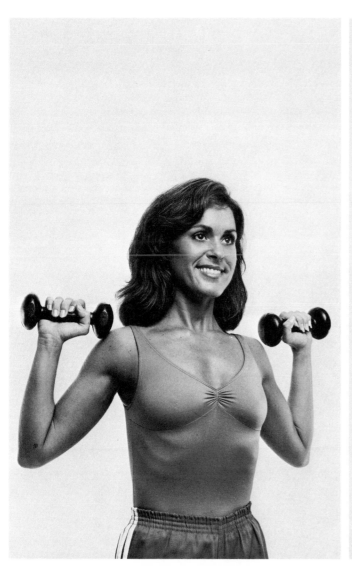
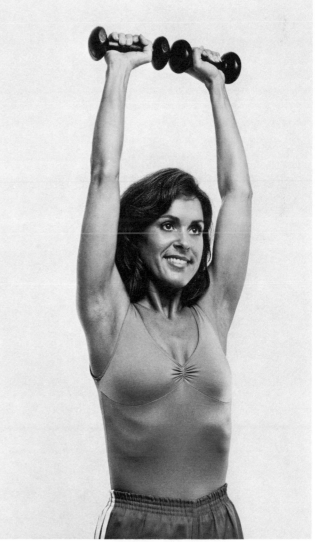

189

ONE-ARM SHOULDER STRETCH

First level: 1 set, 10 sec
Middle level: 2 sets, 15 sec
Top level: 3 sets, 20 sec

Continue doing this exercise exactly as you have been. Be sure that it follows immediately after Dumbbell Press for maximum effect.

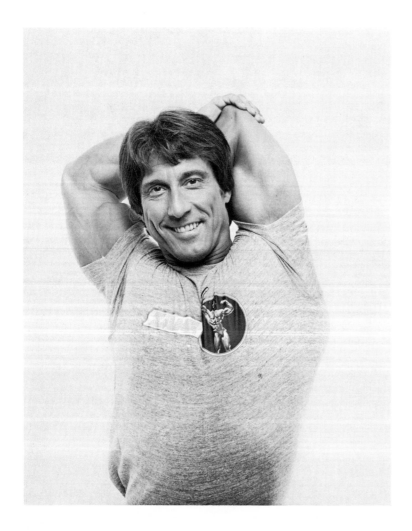

BARBELL FRONT RAISE

First level: 1 set, 10 reps
Middle level: 2 sets, 8 reps
Top level: 3 sets, 12 reps

This is another new exercise, and it really works the front deltoids thoroughly. Stand and grip a barbell in front of you with a distance of 1 foot between each hand. Begin with your arms straight down. Inhale and bring the barbell straight up until it is overhead. Keep your elbows slightly unlocked in this exercise. Exhale as you slowly lower the barbell back to starting position. Repeat.

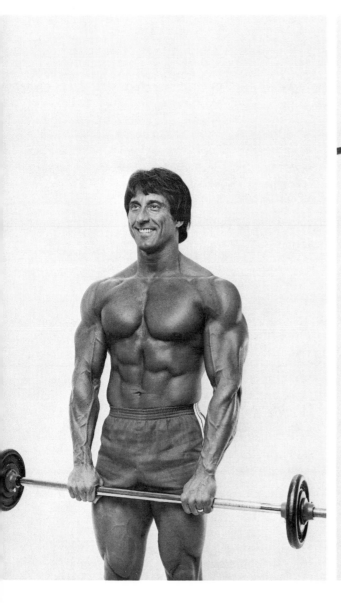
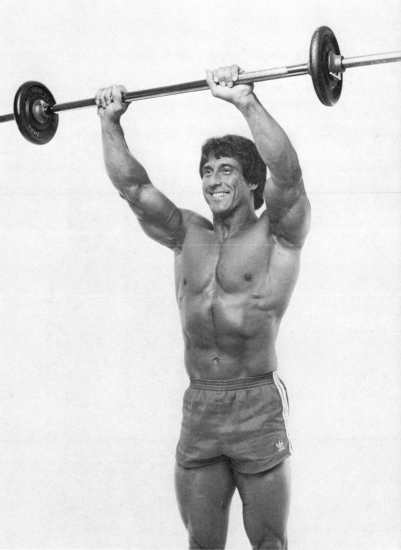

191

DOORKNOB ISOMETRIC FRONT RAISE

First level: 1 set, 10 sec
Middle level: 2 sets, 15 sec
Top level: 3 sets, 20 sec

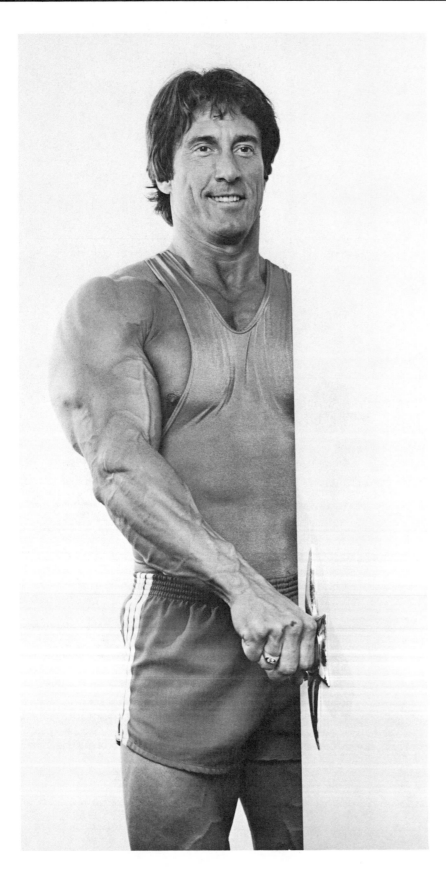

This should be done immediately after Barbell Front Raise. Stand facing a door's edge. Grip the doorknob using an over-hand grip, arms straight, and pull up on the doorknobs with both hands. Hold this tension. Relax. You'll feel this in the front deltoids.

These two exercises improve your appearance when you're standing relaxed!

DUMBBELL SIDE RAISE

First level: 1 set, 10 reps
Middle level: 2 sets, 8 reps
Top level: 3 sets, 12 reps

This movement develops the side or lateral deltoid, which adds width to your shoulders. Lift the dumbbells slowly and feel your deltoids expanding.

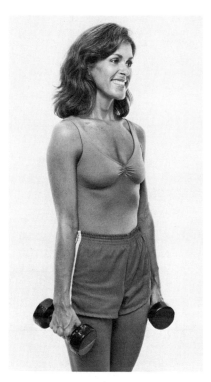
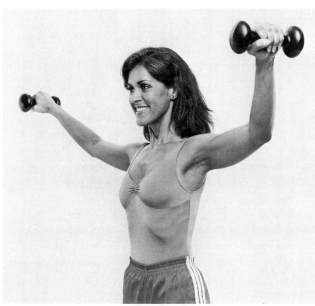

DOORWAY ISOMETRIC LATERAL STRETCH

First level: 1 set, 10 sec
Middle level: 2 sets, 15 sec
Top level: 3 sets, 20 sec

Do this exercise immediately following Dumbbell Side Raise, as you have before. Pushing against an immovable doorway in this way further stimulates the side deltoids.

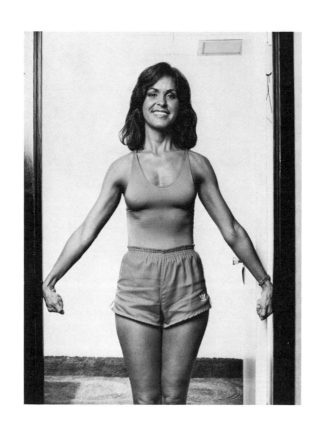

DUMBBELL REAR RAISE

First level: 1 set, 10 reps
Middle level: 2 sets, 8 reps
Top level: 3 sets, 12 reps

DOORWAY ISOMETRIC FRONT STRETCH

First level: 1 set, 10 sec
Middle level: 2 sets, 15 sec
Top level: 3 sets, 20 sec

These should be done immediately following each other as before. This is a great combination to fully stimulate and develop your rear deltoids, a usually neglected and hard-to-work area of the body.

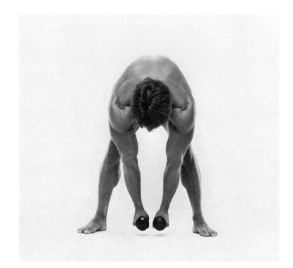
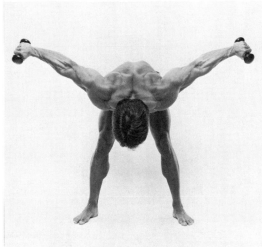

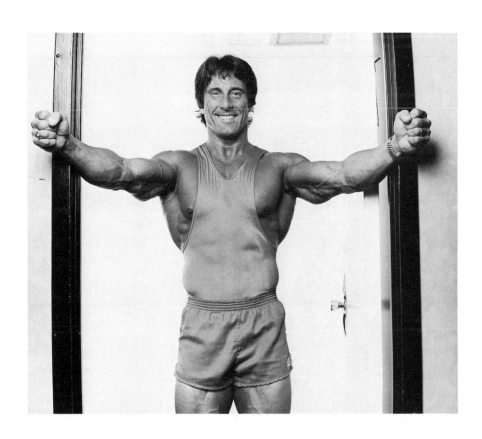

CLOSE-GRIP BENCH PRESS

First level: 1 set, 10 reps
Middle level: 2 sets, 8 reps
Top level: 3 sets, 12 reps

With this exercise, you should be developing a good groove or movement pathway for each repetition. Be sure to keep your elbows out as far from your torso as possible to feel a maximum effect in the outer part of your triceps. Lower the weight slowly to keep in in the groove.

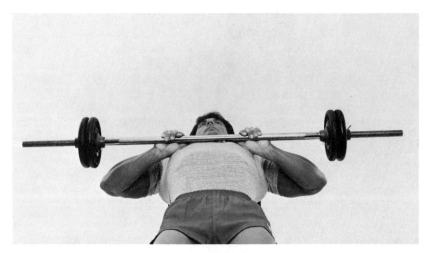

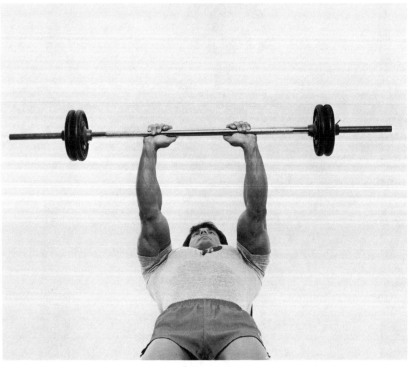

REVERSE DIP STRETCH
BETWEEN CHAIRS

First level: 1 set, 10 sec
Middle level: 2 sets, 15 sec
Top level: 3 sets, 20 sec

Do this stretch the same way as before.
Focus on getting a maximum stretch at
the lowest point.

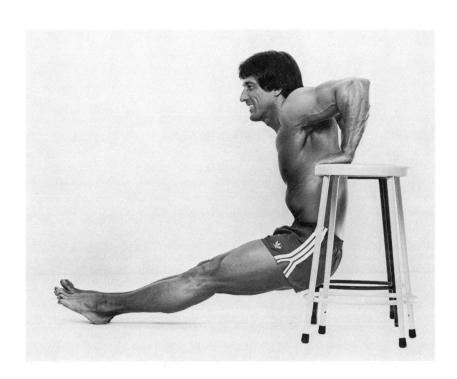

ONE-ARM DUMBBELL EXTENSION

First level: 1 set, 10 reps
Middle level: 2 sets, 8 reps
Top level: 3 sets, 12 reps

Stand and grip a dumbbell in one hand, raise it overhead and bring your elbow in to hug close to your head and slightly back. Inhale and slowly lower the dumbbell until it reaches the back of your neck at the base. Keep your elbow hugging your head throughout this movement. Exhale and slowly extend your arm until almost straight. Repeat. Do this same movement with your other arm. You'll feel the effects mainly in the rear part of your triceps, and you'll get a terrific pump if you allow the dumbbell to stretch down as far as possible.

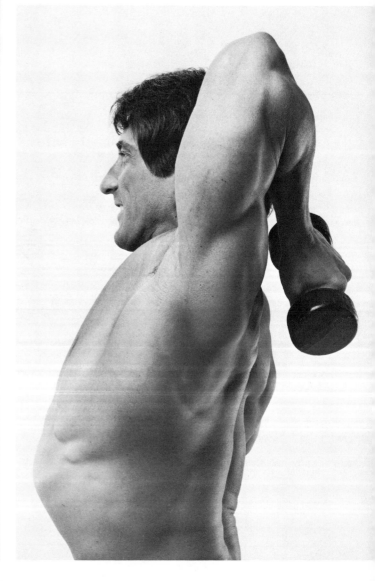

OVERHEAD STRETCH

First level: 1 set, 10 sec
Middle level: 2 sets, 15 sec
Top level: 3 sets, 20 sec

Do this as you did in the Basic Program. By doing this stretch immediately after tricep extensions you'll get the maximum stimulation in the triceps.

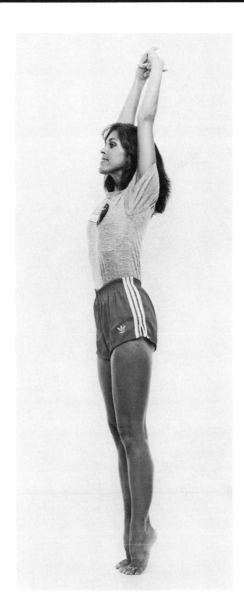

DUMBBELL KICKBACK

First level: 1 set, 10 reps
Middle level: 2 sets, 8 reps
Top level: 3 sets, 12 reps

Holding a dumbbell in each hand, bend over at the waist or lie face down on an incline bench, bring your elbows tight in to your side and push the dumbbells back as far as you can. Hold them in this up position for one second and slowly return them to the starting position. This is an excellent triceps definer and developer. The most important part of the exercise is the contraction, so be sure to straighten your arm out fully. If you hold your upper arms at a 45-degree angle to your sides you'll feel the pump in both rear and lateral (side) sections of your triceps.

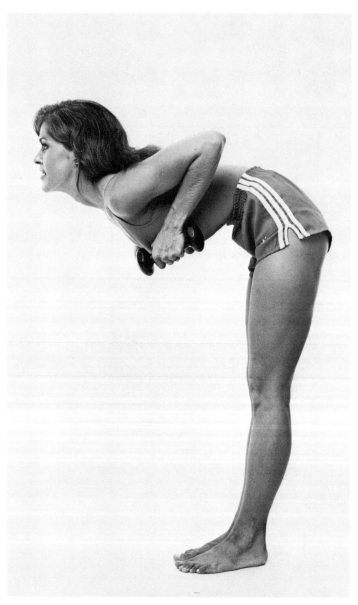
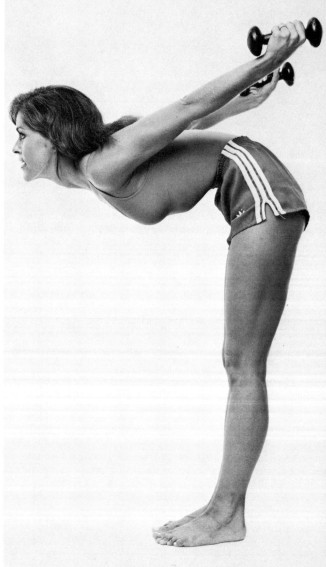

ARMS-BACKWARD STRETCH

First level: 1 set, 10 sec
Middle level: 2 sets, 15 sec
Top level: 3 sets, 20 sec

Do these immediately after the Dumbbell Kickbacks to further stimulate your arms.

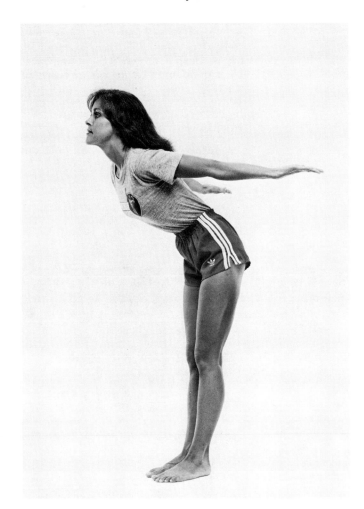

HANGING KNEE-UP

First level: 1 set, 15 reps
Middle level: 2 sets, 20 reps
Top level: 3 sets, 25 reps

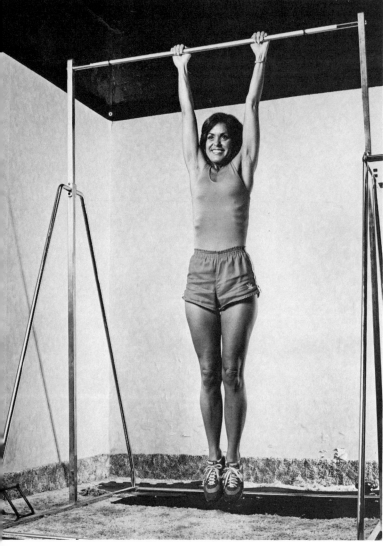

Hang from an overhead bar where your feet clear the floor. Bring your knees up to your chest and return them to a full extension. Exhale as your knees come up, inhale as you lower your legs. This exercise develops the lower abdominals and because it stretches the lower back, it's a good exercise to do in cases of minor soreness in this area. You'll also feel this exercise in the stomach, upper thighs and lower back. Follow with Seated Twist.

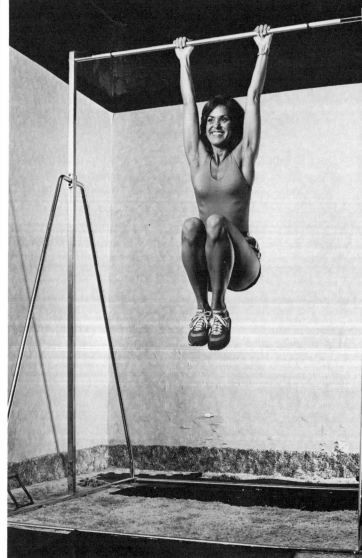

SEATED TWIST

First level: 1 set, 20 reps
Middle level: 2 sets, 25 reps
Top level: 3 sets, 30 reps

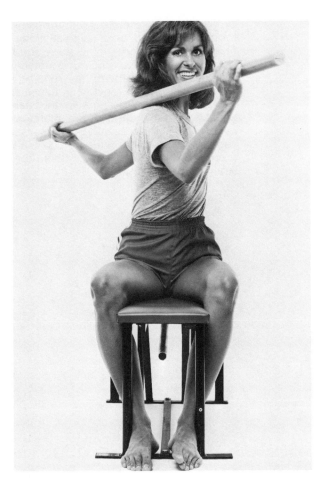

Here is your Day-59 program. This program will also be done on Days 62, 66, 69, 73, 76, 80 and 83.

EXERCISE	Page	First Level	Middle Level	Top Level
One-Leg Top Extension (warm-up)	204	1 set, 30 reps	1 set, 30 reps	1 set, 30 reps
Half Squat	204	1 set, 15 reps	2 sets, 12 reps	3 sets, 18 reps
Lunge on Step	205	1 set, 10 reps	2 sets, 8 reps	3 sets, 12 reps
One-Leg-up Stretch	206	10 seconds	2 sets, 15 sec	3 sets, 20 sec
Leg Curl	207	1 set, 10 reps	2 sets, 8 reps	3 sets, 12 reps
Stiff-Legged Deadlift	208	1 set, 10 reps	2 sets, 8 reps	3 sets, 12 reps
Leg Extension	209	1 set, 10 reps	2 sets, 10 reps	3 sets, 12 reps
Donkey Calf Raise	210	1 set, 30 reps	2 sets, 25 reps	3 sets, 30 reps
Two-Leg Calf Stretch	210	10 seconds	2 sets, 15 sec	3 sets, 20 sec
Standing Calf Raise	211	1 set, 20 reps	2 sets, 15 reps	3 sets, 25 reps
Tibialis Toe Raise	212	1 set, 10 reps	2 sets, 12 reps	3 sets, 15 reps
One-Leg Calf Raise	213	1 set, 15 reps	2 sets, 15 reps	3 sets, 15 reps
Wall Lean (for calves)	213	10 seconds	2 sets, 15 sec	3 sets, 20 sec
Hanging Knee-up	202	1 set, 15 reps	2 sets, 20 reps	3 sets, 25 reps
Bent-Leg Partial Sit-up	214	1 set, 25 reps	2 sets, 30 reps	3 sets, 35 reps
Seated Twist	214	1 set, 25 reps	2 sets, 30 reps	3 sets, 35 reps

ONE-LEG TOP EXTENSION

All levels: 1 set, 20 reps

HALF SQUAT

First level: 1 set, 10 reps
Middle level: 2 sets, 8 reps
Top level: 3 sets, 12 reps

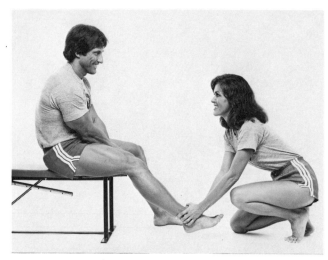

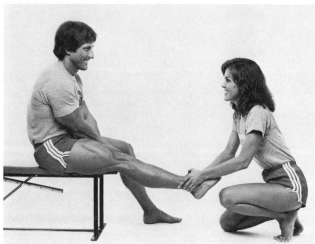

Do your first two exercises with the same form that you have been using all along. Since you have been doing these for a full 8 weeks, you are undoubtedly stronger in both of them; therefore, you will be doing more repetitions for each exercise. Doing high reps in the Half Squat will really stimulate your breathing, so be sure to breathe deeply after each set. You'll also feel the effects of this exercise in the entire thigh, without any strain to your knees.

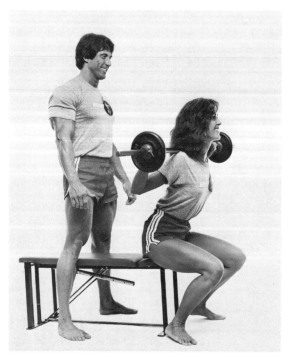

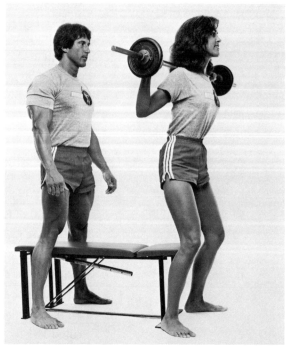

LUNGE ON STEP

First level: 1 set, 10 reps
Middle level: 2sets, 8 reps
Top level: 3 sets, 12 reps

In the Advanced Program we return to this exercise, which you did in the first 4 weeks. Do the Lunge on Step just as you did before and really concentrate on getting into a deep lunge with each repetition. Feel the stimulation to your upper-leg biceps and the outer part of your thighs. This is a full leg developer and you'll feel it in the front of your thighs as well.

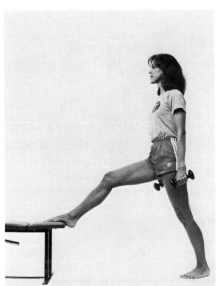
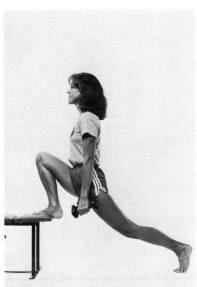

ONE-LEG-UP STRETCH

First level: 1 set, 10 sec
Middle level: 2 sets, 15 sec
Top level: 3 sets, 20 sec

Also do this exercise as you have been doing it before. You're probably discovering that the longer you do this stretch the more the hamstring muscles of the rear thigh loosen up. Your lower back will become more flexible, too, as your head is able to come closer to your knee. If you can already stretch all the way to your knee, touch your chin instead of your forehead.

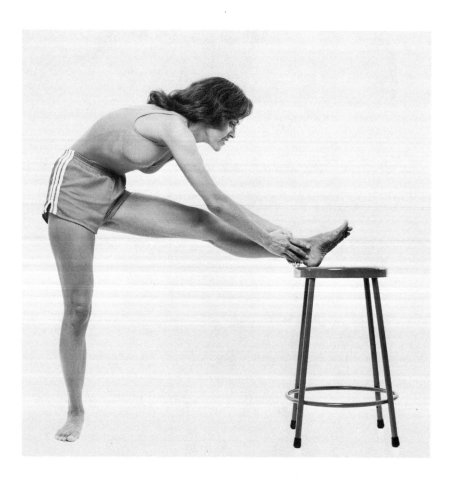

LEG CURL

First level: 1 set, 10 reps
Middle level: 2 sets, 8 reps
Top level: 3 sets, 12 reps

This is an exercise new to the program. You'll need a leg curl machine for this. It works directly on your hamstrings and buttocks. Lie face down on the leg curl table with your knees just off the edge and your ankles under the curling pads. Hold on to each side of the table. (If you don't have access to a leg curl machine, have your partner hold a towel around your ankles and offer resistance.) Inhale and curl your feet and calves up until they touch your buttocks. Hold this position for a moment and then slowly straighten your legs out, lowering the weight, as you exhale.

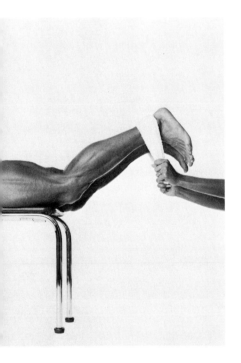

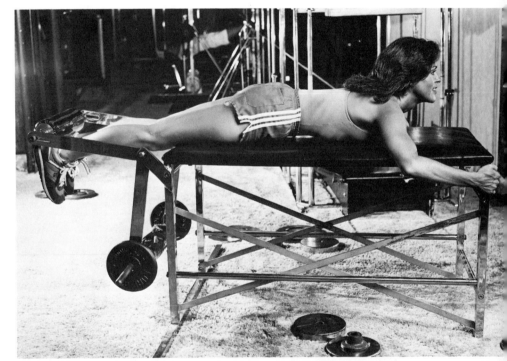

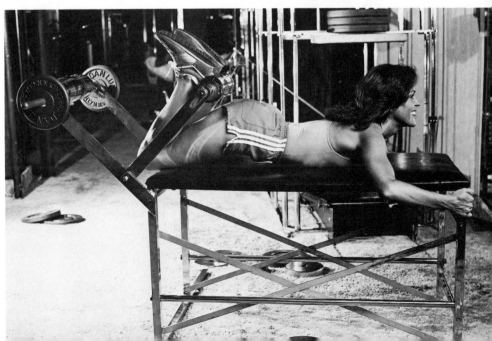

STIFF-LEGGED DEADLIFT

First level: 1 set, 10 reps
Middle level: 2 sets, 8 reps
Top level: 3 sets, 12 reps

You've been doing this exercise for over 5 weeks. The important aspect of this exercise is not how much weight you use but how much of a stretch you get as you go into the bent over, low position. This is excellent to do right after Leg Curls. Leg Curls contract the leg biceps and Stiff-Legged Deadlift stretches them out.

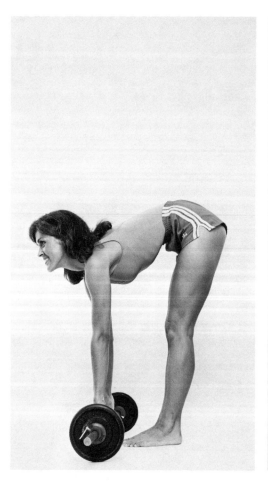
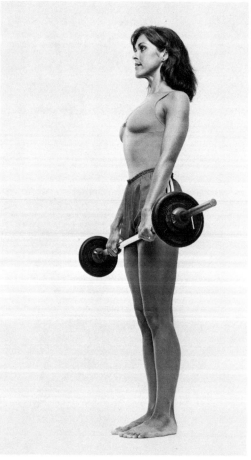

LEG EXTENSION

First level: 1 set, 10 reps
Middle level: 2 sets, 10 reps
Top level: 3 sets, 12 reps

To do this exercise you will need a leg extension table. If you don't have one, you can have your partner apply pressure to the front part of your ankles or attach weights to your legs. This is the best exercise for developing the frontal thighs and strengthening your knees. Sit up on the leg extension table and lean back slightly. Pull yourself back so that your knees are snug against the edge of the table. Put your ankles under the extension pads. Inhale and extend your feet until they are parallel to your thighs. Exhale as you slowly lower the weight to the starting position.

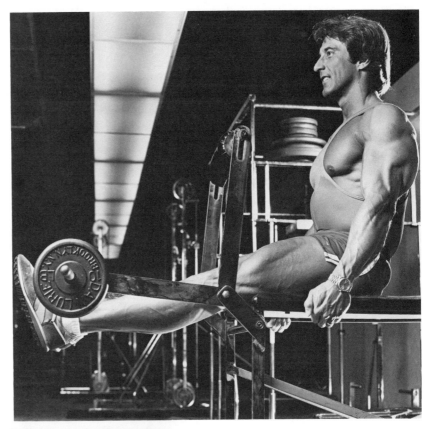

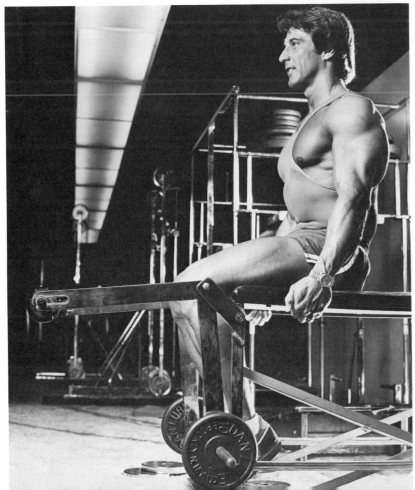

209

DONKEY CALF RAISE

First level: 1 set, 20 reps
Middle level: 2 sets, 15 reps
Top level: 3 sets, 25 reps

TWO-LEG CALF STRETCH

First level: 1 set, 10 sec
Middle level: 2 sets, 15 sec
Top level: 3 sets, 20 sec

Do these in quick succession, as you have been, with one exception. Try holding a little longer at the top of each rep for Donkeys and stretching a little lower for your calves in the Calf Stretch. Visualize your calf muscles expanding as you do each exercise/stretch.

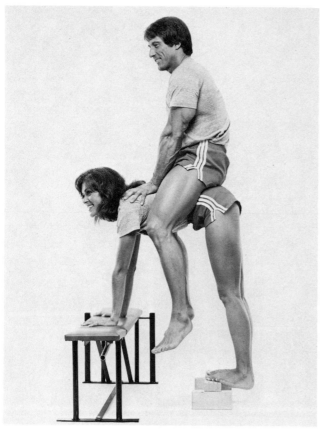

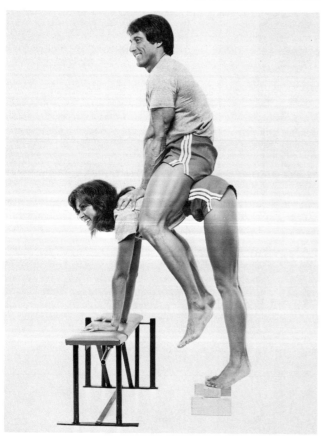

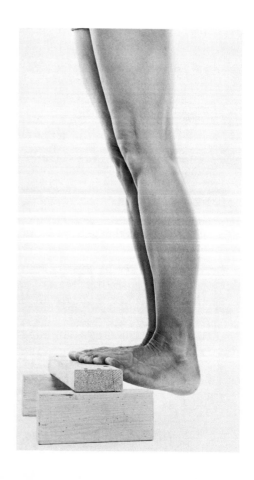

STANDING CALF RAISE

First level: 1 set, 20 reps
Middle level: 2 sets, 15 reps
Top level: 3 sets, 25 reps

You will use a calf machine to do this exercise. If you do not have access to one, substitute Donkey Calf Raise. It is done in the same way as Free-Standing Calf Raise—the only difference being that you have the weight of the calf machine on your shoulders and you are holding on to the calf machine for support. Work for a good pump to your calves instead of using extremely heavy weight.

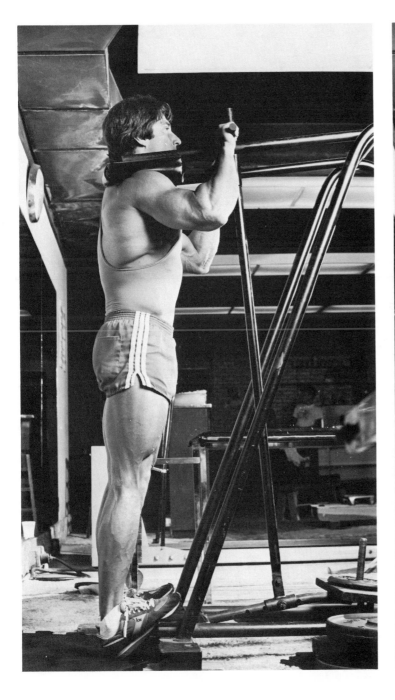
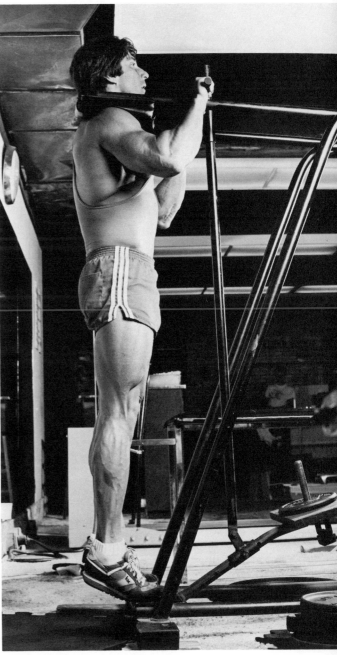

TIBIALIS TOE RAISE

First level: 1 set, 10 reps
Middle level: 2 sets, 12 reps
Top level: 3 sets, 15 reps

This is a good exercise for the front part of your calf, or tibialis (the muscle of the shin area). Stand with your heels on a calf block, lower your toes as much as possible and then raise them as high as possible. Pause a moment in this position, then repeat. Hold on to something or your partner while doing this exercise.

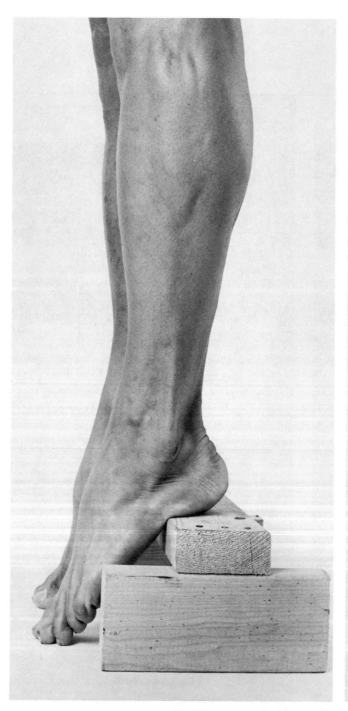
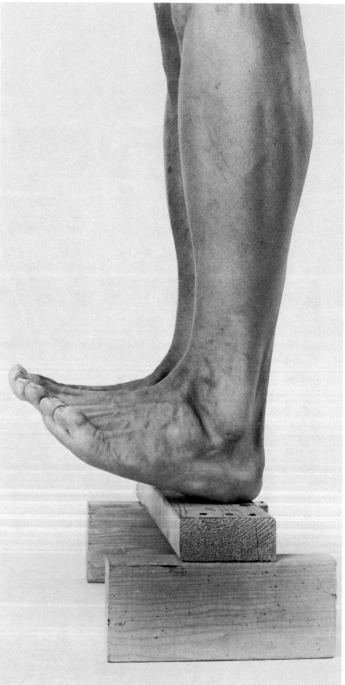

ONE-LEG CALF RAISE

First level: 1 set, 12 reps
Middle level: 2 sets, 15 reps
Top level: 3 sets, 15 reps

WALL LEAN

First level: 1 set, 10 sec
Middle level: 2 sets, 15 sec
Top level: 3 sets, 20 sec

Do these exercises, concentrating on your calves, just as you've been doing them. Notice how strong your ankle and calf muscles have become. For extra stimulation to your calves, pause for a second longer when you reach the highest point in the One-Leg Calf Raise.

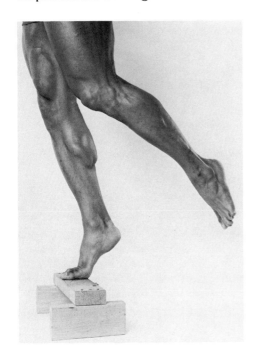

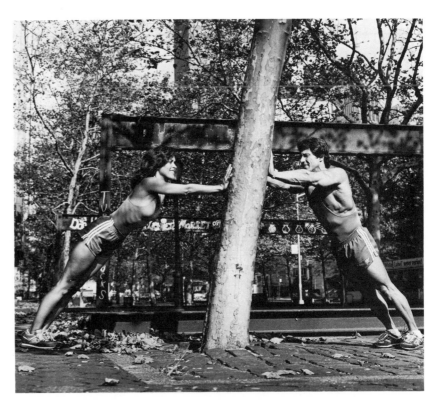

BENT-LEG PARTIAL SIT-UP

First level: 1 set, 20 reps
Middle level: 2 sets, 25 reps
Top level: 3 sets, 30 reps

SEATED TWIST

First level: 1 set, 20 reps
Middle level: 2 sets, 25 reps
Top level: 3 sets, 30 reps

Do these as you've been doing them, but with slightly higher repetitions for each set. Or do all the reps from all the sets in one set!

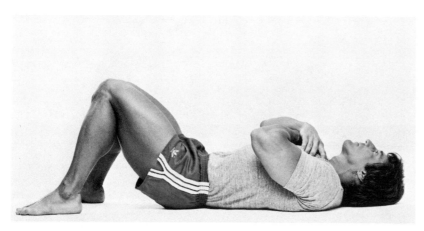

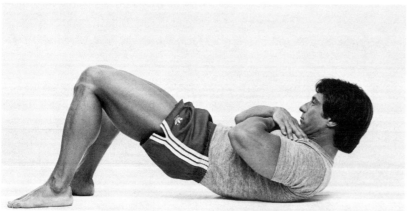

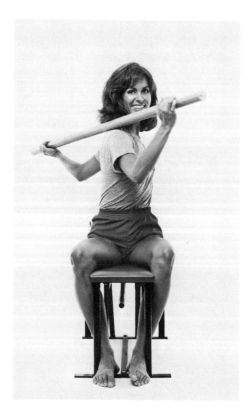

DAILY ADVANCED PROGRAM
Weeks 9 to 12

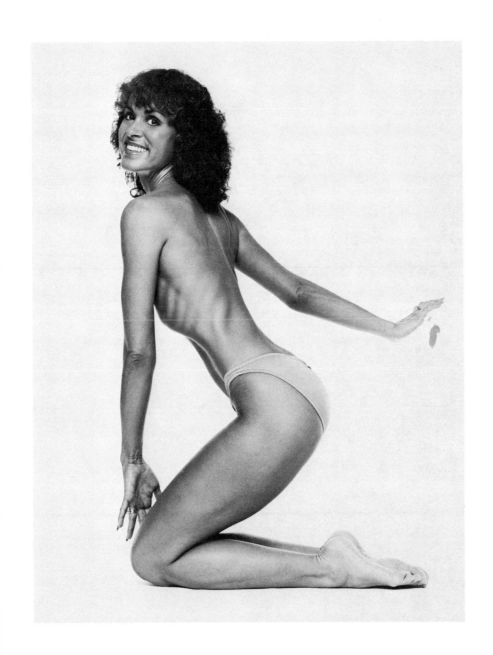

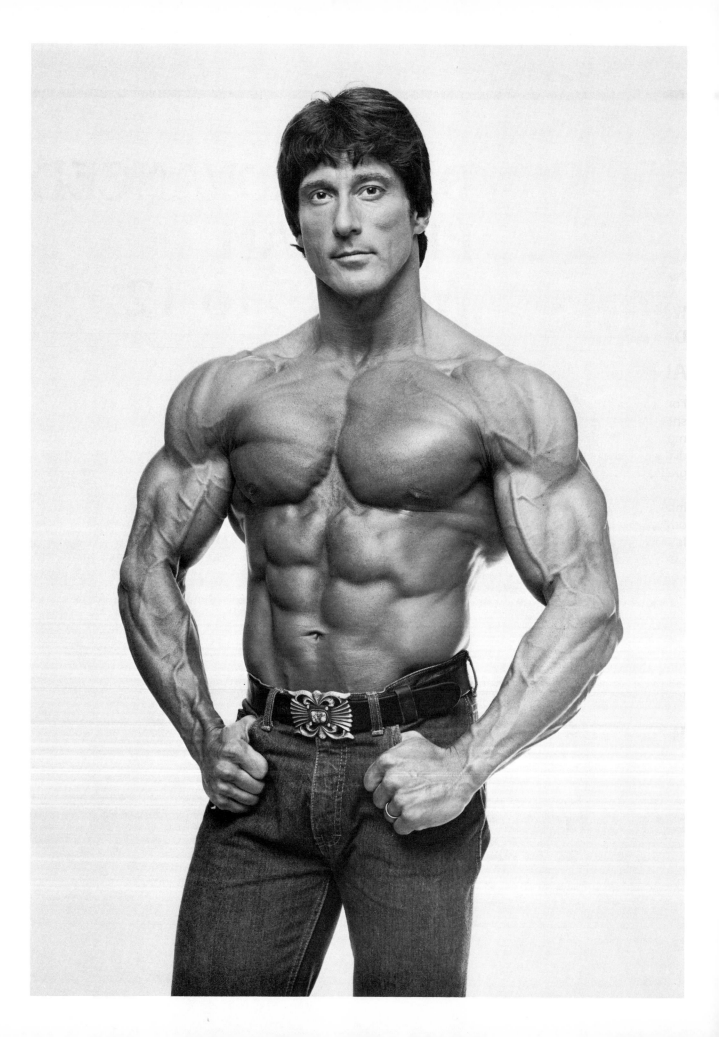

Week Nine
Day 57

AEROBIC EXERCISE

For the next 4 weeks we will be making fewer comments about what you should be doing in your exercise program, in the hope that you will develop more self-direction. We do recommend reading over the Basic and Intermediate Programs when you can, to refresh your memory and keep you progressing toward your goal.

Your aerobic exercises will begin with 3 minutes and increase in 30-second intervals, instead of 15-second intervals as before. If you aren't doing any other daily aerobic work like swimming, jogging, running, cycling or any fast-paced exercise for a sustained period of time, or even if you are doing extra aerobics, you shoud regard the times that we suggest as the minimum, not the maximum. If you do decide to increase your time, do it gradually. Use the same pattern for increasing the time that was outlined in the previous programs. Don't limit yourself if you are capable of more. Strive for the ultimate!

Your time for Quick Paced Step-ups today is 3 minutes. This will be our final reminder to warm up and warm down properly. The more time you spend doing the exercise, the more time you need to warm down. Have fun, be happy and think positively!

WEIGHT TRAINING AND STRETCHING

Today is the first day of your new Advanced Program. This section will take you a little longer to complete because it contains more exercises and stretches. These additional movements work the back, biceps, forearms and waist from many different angles, giving you a more complete development.

Suppose your partner is following the program at a different level than you are? If this is the case, the person at the higher level always does his/her set first. This allows partners at the first and middle levels to set a good pace without wasting time. The same is true for partners working at the middle and top levels. A first-level person should not work with a top-level person because the former would have to wait too long between sets, thus lessening the effectiveness of the first-level program.

ADVANCED DIET TIP

Prepare a special meal for your partner this week. Use your food almanac to choose foods high in nutrition and low in carbohydrates and calories. Spend as little time in preparation as possible. Serve a good variety of foods from the various food groups. Be aware of the textures and colors; and display the food artistically. For dessert, serve a fresh fruit which complements the meal. You'll find a lot of suggestions in the recipe section. Whatever you serve, the dessert should be light and small. Allow your partner to help you prepare the food. We like to work together in the kitchen because the preparation time seems to go more quickly and the work is much more enjoyable. When you sit down to eat you know that you have both contributed to the meal, and that is a very good feeling. If you can't get together to cook, meet somewhere for lunch and share foods that you have each prepared ahead of time. Ask your partner what he/she prefers to eat, or prepare something as a surprise dish. This is a way to encourage each other to stay on a healthy diet and is a lot of fun besides. Sometimes when you are cutting back on certain foods and carbohydrates it's difficult to choose the right foods for yourself. If you allow someone else to make the selections for you (especially when you are feeling weak willed) you will find it easier to remain on your healthful eating

If the day on which you decide to share a meal with your partner is your rest day from exercising, remember that you won't be doing as much physically and therefore should choose a meal that is smaller, lighter and lower in fats and carbohydrates. Choose foods that are easily digested. Prepare something special and different from the ordinary fare you are accustomed to having. Be creative! And be sure to keep careful records of what you eat.

Preparing and eating nutritious food is rewarding. You derive personal satisfaction from the creation of the meal, oral gratification from the pure and natural tastes of the food, and a sense of achievement from the increasing improvement of your body's shape, tone, appearance and stamina. Prepare the meal for your partner and yourself with awareness and loving care. It will be appreciated.

Day 58

AEROBIC EXERCISE

You will notice that now you're breathing more easily than ever before during your physical activities. If you increase the time spent in your aerobic exercises you will also increase your breathing capacity. Your aerobic time for today is 3 minutes and 30 seconds of Quick Paced Step-ups.

WEIGHT TRAINING AND STRETCHING

You may be training with a partner whose strength is very different from yours. For example, Frank normally does Bench Press for 10 reps with 235 pounds while Christine usually uses 60 pounds for 10 reps. We feel the exercises as we are supposed to because we are using as much weight as we can for the designated reps as we pursue our different goals. So don't worry if you're not using the same weights as your partner. That's why weight-training equipment is adjustable. Doing the exercise correctly and feeling it in the appropriate areas is much more important than the amount of weight you use.

Day 59

AEROBIC EXERCISE

If you do aerobic work that entails using your feet a great deal—like jogging, walking or running—we advise that you spare no expense and buy proper shoes. Good equipment will pay for itself many times over. It lasts longer and can even help prevent injuries. This is especially true of proper shoes. Check with an athletic-shoe specialist to help you choose the correct shoes for your sport. Another point to remember is: Never buy any equipment unless you are going to use it. Just because you have paid for some kind of gear and it is sitting in plain view every day does not mean that you will benefit just from looking at it! Wear a good pair of jogging shoes if you have them. You will get a great deal more spring in your Step-ups. Your aerobic time for today is 4 minutes of Quick Paced Step-ups.

WEIGHT TRAINING AND STRETCHING

Today is the first day of your leg and waist exercises in the Advanced Program. These may seem a little easier to do than any of the upper-body programs you've been doing the last two days, because there are fewer exercises and stretches involved. Nevertheless, the thighs are the biggest muscle group in the body and consequently take more energy to work. So don't let up; just move right through these exercises as you did in your other programs. Your workout should not be a contest between you and your partner to see who can lift the most weight; You should continue to use heavier and heavier weights only if you want your muscles to grow. So if your aim is to stay slim and well toned, use the lighter weights (those recommended in the Intermediate Program) and rest less between sets. You can attain excellent shape and development by using light weights if you make sure to do each exercise correctly and feel the increased circulation in your muscles.

Day 60

AEROBIC EXERCISE

Did you ever question why you need both aerobic and anaerobic forms of exercise? (So often people seem to do either one or the other.) We believe that these two types of exercise complement each other. If you only do exercises for your muscles and tendons (anaerobic) and develop a beautiful outer appearance, what about your inner beauty? It's like having a car with no engine! What good is that? The opposite is also true. If you only condition your organs and don't do anything for what holds you together, what good is that? An engine with no chassis is going nowhere unless it's part of a complete automobile—one with both a well-tuned engine and a strong, sleek chassis. And, of course, the rewards are all yours when you have this much going for you! A beautiful, healthy, strong body!

Your time today for the aerobic Step-ups is 4 minutes and 30 seconds.

WEIGHT TRAINING AND STRETCHING

Do you have any muscular soreness from the last three days' workouts? Where is it? Soreness is often an indication of which exercises are working your body parts the hardest. Can you figure out the exercises that are causing the soreness? Today in your workout, pay special attention to where you feel the stimulation after you complete each exercise. This way you'll develop personal, first-hand knowledge about each exercise and your reaction to it. Today you repeat Day 57.

Day 61

AEROBIC EXERCISE

You are doing sensationally! Keep it up! Set your timer for 5 minutes today and begin your Quick Paced Step-ups.

WEIGHT TRAINING AND STRETCHING

Today repeat the Day-58 program. Pay attention to exactly where you feel the pump/stimulation from each exercise.

Day 62

AEROBIC EXERCISE

If you're tense before you begin your warm-ups, don't push it. You will only have more difficulty relaxing. Instead, take a few minutes to sit down in a quiet place and begin breathing very deeply and exhaling completely. Close your eyes and count each breath you take. Place your full attention on your breath. This technique will help release the tension and ready you for your warm-up. Tension tends to decrease flexibility. So unless you loosen up first, working your muscles may cause them to become even tighter and more tense and inflexible. This can cause injuries. Set your timer for 5 minutes and 30 seconds today, for Quick Paced Step-ups.

WEIGHT TRAINING AND STRETCHING

Repeat Day 59 today.

Day 63

AEROBIC EXERCISE, WEIGHT TRAINING AND STRETCHING

Today is your rest day. You've completed the first week in the Advanced Program and you're very close to realizing your goal. Do some reading or go see a movie today. Choose something inspirational.

MUTUAL-ASSISTANCE TECHNIQUE

Offer to give your partner a massage. Does he/she have any sore areas? Take turns massaging each other. Neck, shoulders, upper and lower back, arms and upper chest, waist, hips and legs as well as feet should be massaged. Read our section on massage.

BODY AWARENESS

Today is the best time to take another set of "before" photos. Take the same views at the same time of day and at the same distance from the camera as you remember doing back on Day 29. Get these photos developed as soon as possible. Again request 8-by-10 shots of your 4 views—front, left side, back, right side. Color photos and slides are most helpful.

Without the use of a mirror or photos, draw from memory and to the best of your ability a picture of the way you think you look—now that you have made so much progress in your training and nutritional programs.

In a quiet, comfortable place stand with your eyes closed. Visualize yourself as a silhouette or a shadow. In your mind's eye, carefully inspect all the subtleties of your silhouette. Have your silhouette turn and view it from both sides and back. Inspect each view carefully. See every detail. When you have done this from all sides of your body, form an overall view of yourself, and give yourself a positive compliment about how you look. Date a new page in the Body Awareness section of your journal, and write your feelings about all the awareness exercises you have just done. Write down anything that pertains to your becoming more aware of your body, including your emotional response to what has been happening to you.

Week Ten
Day 64

AEROBIC EXERCISE

Today we return to High Kicks. While you are doing the High Kicks, get a clear image in your mind of exactly how you look doing the movement. You should feel as though you're standing to one side and watching yourself. Your aerobic time for today is 3 minutes.

WEIGHT TRAINING AND STRETCHING

Did you have a good day of relaxation yesterday? Today you start back on the Day-57 program. Your rests between sets should be averaging between 1 and 1½ minutes. As you get better and better at this Advanced Program, rest less and less. Eventually you'll be able to take only 1-minute rests.

ADVANCED DIET TIP

When shopping for food, choose carefully. Just because you may have purchased something in a health food store doesn't necessarily mean it's good for you. We have found a great many health food stores stocked with health-junk foods. Most of the candy bars, cakes, cookies, flavored yogurts, packaged snacks, and frozen yogurts are loaded with sugar! If you have a problem with your blood sugar, and your moods fluctuate all through the day (especially after eating) you should be avoiding these foods. Your body gets a very small amount of minerals and vitamins from the sweeteners used in these products (such as honey, fructose and raw sugar). You can get more vitamins and minerals from other sources without the calories and without shooting your blood sugar up so quickly. Read all the labels on the food before you purchase it. Your body is going to treat all sugars the same way. Unless they are used up immediately, they will be stored as fat in places like your stomach, waistline, thighs and upper arms. When you're getting plenty of protein, vegetables (both raw and cooked), some fats and some fruits, you won't crave sweet things. In fact, you'll reeducate your taste buds so that when you do eat something with added sweetener, you won't enjoy it. It will seem too sweet. You might think that substituting artificial sweeteners will safely satisfy your cravings and cause no problems. This may be a mistake for you, as it is for most people: Artificial sweeteners can perpetuate instead of satisfying your craving for sweets. These additives can trigger insulin secretion as well, shooting your blood sugar up just as if you'd eaten sugar —with a resultant weight gain. If sweets are the main problem food in your diet and you've tried many times to give them up entirely and still haven't succeeded, then give them up gradually. In this way you will hardly notice their absence. But there must come a time when sweets are no longer a part of your diet. Start by not sweetening your beverages. Then continue to slowly eliminate sugar from other foods you eat. If you must replace it do so with fresh fruit in small amounts—but be sure to check their caloric and carbohydrate content. Start paying closer attention to what is in your food. You will feel more and more fantastic as a result!

Day 65

AEROBIC EXERCISE

When your abdomen is strong, your lower back becomes stronger. High Kicks work on these two areas. A lot of injuries occur when people are performing simple tasks, and usually the problem is in the lower back. If your back is strong and reinforced by well-developed abdominals, these injuries will be less likely to occur. Warm up your back today by doing some seated stretches. Sit on the floor and hold your feet in a flexed position. Gradually stretch your hands out to reach your toes. Grasp your big toes, with each index finger used as a hook. Slowly bring your head to your knees without straining or bouncing. Relax into the stretch and hold for 10 seconds. Relax and repeat.

Your aerobic time today is 3 full minutes of High Kicks.

WEIGHT TRAINING AND STRETCHING

When you exercise today, exercise for yourself, but keep in mind that you are also setting an example for others to follow. If you have children and they see how dedicated you are to keeping a healthy, fit body, in most cases they will begin to imitate you at some stage. This can apply not only to children, but to other family members, friends and acquaintances as well. When they see you getting in shape and feeling "on top of it" all the time, they will want to know your secret and they will begin to listen to you. Someone who preaches fitness but doesn't follow his own advice is not going to be taken very seriously. We have had more success by setting a good example than by trying to verbally convince everyone of the benefits of regular exercise. People want to know secrets. They see something, and they want to have it. Continue setting a good example for those around you. Be concerned with your progress and others will become concerned with theirs. This attitude will have a beneficial effect on both you and your partner.

Today you will repeat Day 58. Because you are doing more exercise for each body part, you're shaping up much faster. Keep noticing these improvements as they occur.

Day 66

AEROBIC EXERCISE

Exercise, and especially hard exercise like aerobic work, can help protect you from becoming overweight. If you are active, you digest your food more efficiently; it moves more quickly through your digestive system, thereby decreasing the absorption of excess food energy. The longer the food stays in your body, the more unneeded calories are absorbed and stored as fat. You use more of your food and burn more calories when you exercise. Therefore you can afford to eat just a little more than you could if you weren't exercising. You'll also find that you don't have cravings and feel constantly hungry. If you cut back on your exercising, cut back on your caloric intake. It's as simple as that.

Your aerobic time for High Kicks today is 4 minutes.

WEIGHT TRAINING AND STRETCHING

Repeat the Day-59 program. When working your legs today, go for maximum pump/stimulation in each area. This is the way to make progress and beneficial changes in short periods. Make every set really count.

Day 67

AEROBIC EXERCISE

We can never stress too much the benefits of aerobics for your heart and circulatory system. Heart disease and high blood pressure can be prevented and even eliminated through proper exercise. Aerobics help to do this by lowering the pulse and blood pressure, relaxing your body and relieving stress and tension. Everyone experiences some degree of stress every day. But you can eliminate it every day by exercising!

Your time for High Kick aerobics today is 4 minutes and 30 seconds.

WEIGHT TRAINING AND STRETCHING

Repeat the Day-57 program. The stimulation that a pump gives you always means progress. Often it's better not to keep increasing the weights but to stick to the weight that gives you the most stimulation. The heavier the weight, the harder it is to do the exercise correctly. Don't sacrifice form and a good pump for more weight. The pump is beneficial in terms of health because it causes the blood to rush through your body carrying nutrients to aid the muscle that you're exercising.

Day 68

AEROBIC EXERCISE

A great many athletes in strength sports build up their bodies to the point of being overweight but not fat. They need these extra pounds to enable them to handle more weight and be stronger. Football players, weight lifters, power lifters, and shot-putters are all in this category. In fact, compared with the average person, they probably have less fat and a lot more muscle for the size of their frame. Most athletes or fitness advocates are easily spotted:

Their bodies don't have any bulges or bumps. Combat unsightly lumps and bumps of ugly fat on your body—exercise!

Today your aerobic High Kick time is 5 minutes.

WEIGHT TRAINING AND STRETCHING

Repeat your Day-58 program today. As you're getting into better and better shape, you're probably noticing that people are treating you differently. We know that our physical presence is more dynamic and we command more respect when we are in top shape. The fact that people notice your physical condition will inspire confidence in you. There is no greater incentive to keeping in shape and exercising regularly than having your progress noticed by others. Keep up the good work by training hard today!

Day 69

AEROBIC EXERCISE

Did you know that on the average most of us spend over half of an entire year indoors and inactive? Unless we are lucky and our jobs allow us to get outside often, we are missing a lot of fresh air and sunshine. If the weather is good and the environment is safe, exercise outdoors. You'll breathe more clearly in the fresh air, and the sunshine always feels great. We definitely feel stronger when we exercise outside. Just be sure that the weather is not overly hot, cold or smoggy. Enjoy yourself. Pamper your body, bathe it in sunshine and fresh air!

The time for aerobic High Kicks today is 5 minutes and 30 seconds.

WEIGHT TRAINING AND STRETCHING

For today's workout, repeat the program for Day 59. How do your legs feel in relation to the rest of your body? Everybody has some areas that respond more slowly than others. These are "weak points." If your legs are your weak point, then do an extra set of 2 or 3 exercises or stretches that are the most beneficial to this lagging area.

Day 70

AEROBIC EXERCISE, WEIGHT TRAINING AND STRETCHING

Today is your rest day, so indulge in a relaxing activity. Do some sunbathing, if possible, or swim to loosen and stretch your body. Or get into a hot tub or Whirlpool hydro-massage and then take a sauna for ultimate relaxation. You've completed 10 weeks, so pamper yourself.

MUTUAL-ASSISTANCE TECHNIQUE

Having faith in your ability to reach your goals is essential for progress. If you are 100 percent certain of success, then you'll reach your goals even faster. Since you know you'll win, learn to behave as if you already have. We don't mean being arrogant and acting as if you know everything. Always balance a positive attitude with humility and be willing to accept advice and criticism.

BODY AWARENESS

Have available your "before" photos which were taken on Day 35 and the photos you took on Day 63. Date the Day-63 photos. Lay these photos down side by side and study all the changes that have occurred in the 4-week period. You'll notice that your weak areas are coming closer to what you see as your goal, and that other areas of your body which weren't of such great concern are really beginning to enhance your overall look. Spend at least 20 minutes studying the photos. Try to view this body as though it isn't yours, but someone else's. For every one thing that you still consider a challenge, find two things that are positive assets.

Using eight sheets of tracing paper, trace the outline of your body on the photos from Days 35 and 63. Compare these tracings carefully and mentally note the changes in your body.

In an advanced program you will often experience more soreness. Sit in a quiet place where you are comfortable and will not be disturbed. Concentrate on a sore area of your body. Visualize this area very deeply beneath the surface. See it becoming very white and warm, until the warmth and color spread and engulf the entire sore spot. Now imagine the soreness as a white cloud. See the cloud lift away from your body and float away. The soreness is gone. Do this with all your sore areas. Be sure that the cloud picks up all the soreness and removes it totally.

Date a clean page in the Body Awareness section of your journal and write about your experiences with the awareness exercise today.

Week Eleven
Day 71

AEROBIC EXERCISE

If you have a particularly difficult time getting warmed up, here is a technique that we use when this happens to us or when we want to cut corners on cold mornings. Take a shower or bath! If you soak or stand in a warm bath or shower for 5 or 10 minutes, your muscles will begin loosening up and will make your warm-ups easier. Don't make the water too hot or it will exhaust you; just have it comfortably warm. Get your entire body wet, including your head. Use a brush or loofah to stimulate circulation. Your body will feel alive and glowing after sloughing off all the dead skin, and you'll feel full of energy and pep.

Your aerobic time for Jump Rope today is 3 minutes.

WEIGHT TRAINING AND STRETCHING

Repeat your Day-57 program today. Really put a lot into your training sessions this week. You are halfway through the Advanced Program and well accustomed to each exercise, so work on the intensity factor in your sessions. Keep aiming at doing more work in less time, on each set and within each repetition. Try to keep up this intensity all week and make it a new, positive habit for you.

ADVANCED DIET TIP

We've always felt that eating at home is the most delicious and nutritious way to dine. We prefer to use the extra money we would have spent at a restaurant (for tax, tips, valet service and convenience) to buy high-quality food that can be prepared nutritiously, and with loving care, at home. Eating this way gives us more privacy and enjoyment—plus it's money spent wisely.

For many reasons, however, it isn't always possible to eat at home. We travel a great deal, and are forever finding ourselves in a city where the choice is fast-foods or room service. Often after arriving home from a trip there is no food in the house, so we go out to eat for the sake of convenience. And like everyone else, occasionally we go out to eat just for a change of environment and to relax and enjoy ourselves. Whatever the reason for eating out, we always find ourselves faced with the challenge of where and what to eat.

When you decide to eat out, choose a restaurant that serves high-quality protein meals and fresh vegetables. We watch the delivery trucks that pull up outside restaurants early in the day, and make mental notes for future reference. We avoid those with all the pre-cut, frozen food trucks outside! Stay away from any restaurant that has that mouth-watering dessert you just can't resist. Many of our favorite restaurants don't even offer desserts (thank heaven); but of course there are those that serve fresh-baked, whole-grain breads and desserts, which we stay away from as long as we are working toward a goal. It's a lot easier to resist fattening foods if you avoid them completely. Before you go to a restaurant, call ahead and see if they serve the foods that you prefer. We always call and ask what their main courses are, if they serve fresh vegetables, fresh fruits and cheeses . . . all naturally and without sauces.

When you choose a restaurant, look for a health food or deli type of establishment. When you eat foods like Italian (too much salt, sauces and starches), Chinese (sauces, additives like MSG and sugar), Japanese (MSG, flour, sugar) and Mexican (starches and sauces), you get a lot more than you actually want for a healthy diet. These additions are often "hidden" and can greatly add up in terms of calories and carbohydrates.

Just because you happen to be in a health food restaurant doesn't mean you can safely eat anything on the menu. Stay away from honey-laden foods, yogurts that are frozen or flavored (contain additives and sweeteners) and any of the food that could be too starchy for your diet. In deli-style restaurants, stay away from the spicy, cured foods, noodles and other heavy starches. As far as fast-foods are concerned, we don't even consider these to be food. The stuff that they serve at fast-food chains has been subjected to every method you can imagine to destroy most of the nutrients that were there at the beginning. Fast-foods have been frozen, overheated, heavily salted, and sugared, spiced, boiled and broiled with rancid oil and fats (you can smell them before you arrive at the establishment); and if they have salads (by far the safest thing to order), remember that the ingredients could have been cut up days ago! Stop at a grocery store for fresh fruit and cheese, or fresh raw vegetables, and some milk, instead of going to a fast-food place. Carry some canned tuna (water packed) with you for emergencies.

Usually appetizers served at restaurants contain "extras" and too many calories. Next time you order the first course, choose it to suit your needs. For example, if you order a shrimp or crab cocktail, request that they omit the sauce and bring a wedge of lime or lemon instead (or even a little melted butter). Tomato juice with celery sticks, grapefruit half, melon and meat appetizers are good choices also. Sometimes we can't find anything decent to order on the menu, or the appetizers sound better than the main courses, so we order our dinner from the appetizers. These can be chopped liver, rumaki, mushrooms, raw vegetables, fish cocktails (without the sauce) or melon. Then we can order a salad and are pretty well satisfied, more so than if we'd eaten something we really didn't want, and had to suffer from indigestion for the rest of the day.

Soups, even if they say homemade, can be full of extras. They generally are oversalted and contain sugar. Chefs think this brings out the flavor of the soup. We think if the food had flavor in the first place, you wouldn't need to coax it out with all the additions. If you keep these things in mind when you are in a restaurant, your meal can be enjoyable not only while you're eating, but also later—when you are free of dyspeptic aftereffects.

As we said, in a restaurant your safest choice of food is usually the salad. Of course it could be pre-cut and could have lost some nutrients through oxidation, but it will have lost less than any overcooked, pre-cut food. Always ask for your dressing to be served on the side. If you don't, the salad can really be smothered beyond recognition! Plain oil and vinegar or lemon wedges are the best dressing you can use. Most restaurants use bottled dressing, and even if they make their own it probably contains salt, sugar and/or honey. Don't bother asking if the food contains salt or sweetening; most likely they don't know what's in it. Sugar is sometimes added to vegetables, whether fresh or not. So if you really want to be safe in a place you're not particularly sure of, stick to a salad or fresh fruit and cottage cheese as your side dish. Can you imagine how many extra calories and carbohydrates you're getting when you eat in a restaurant?

We've told you about all the sugar and salt in the vegetables and soups. What about the main course? Can you trust it? Unless it's a broiled steak, fish without breading or baked plain, probably not. Yes, they even put sugar in meats. You'll find this especially true at buffet-style restaurants, where you can eat all you want (or all you can stomach!). Sugar is used as a preservative and a flavor enhancer. Choose meats without gravies, sauces and breading or batters. You can request your food without all the extras; and if you prefer, some restaurants will even serve your food broiled instead of fried. Always request that your food be unsalted. Along with your main course generally comes a choice of rice or potato. Skip this entirely and have it left off your plate (too tempting in some cases). Early in the day this rice or potato could make an entire meal in itself. Add a little lemon and a touch of butter to your meat and have some cheese or fresh tomatoes along with your meal.

For your beverage skip the coffee and tea unless they serve herb tea. You could bring your own herb tea if you like. Chamomile is a very good after-dinner tea, because it's an aid to digestion. Most restaurants carry natural spring water, or you can order club soda with a twist of lime or lemon. This is a very clean and refreshing drink. Milk is an excellent choice for those who want to gain weight and for those whose system can tolerate it.

Alcohol can be a poison if drunk in large amounts. But taken in small quantities it can help stimulate your appetite, speed up and assist digestion, and induce relaxation and drowsiness. Light beers, which are low in calories and carbohydrates (limit one or two 12-ounce bottles a day), are best for this purpose. Dry red, rosé and white wines (white is lowest in calories) should be taken in smaller amounts (limit: half a bottle to 12 ounces daily). These limits vary among individuals, according to size and age. We are not advocating drinking alcohol if you don't do so already. We are just suggesting some guidelines for those who find giving it up difficult.

If you're often tempted to have dessert in a restaurant, maybe you aren't getting enough to eat. Or maybe you're eating out of desire and habit rather than hunger. If you insist on ending your meal with something special, have fresh fruit with a little cheese; however, don't have fruit and cheese for dessert if you had it during the meal. You don't want to overdo it. Order a cheese tray and share it with others. Skip the bread and crackers that generally come with the order and see if you can get a few sticks of fresh raw vegetables instead. This way you won't have to use your will power. Eat only small amounts and very slowly. Remember, you just ate a full and satisfying meal, and it takes time for your stomach to register "full." When you're enjoying yourself and engaged in conversation, unless you are really careful, you could overeat. Always leave the table satisfied but not stuffed. Leave with a pleasant feeling.

Day 72

AEROBIC EXERCISE

Your time for Jump Rope today is 3 minutes and 30 seconds. If you ever get a pain in your side from doing too much, too soon, slow down your movements. If the pain continues, bend forward at the waist, place your hands on your knees and exhale through your mouth. Without taking a breath, pull in your stomach to form a vacuum. Massage the area where there is pain very gently with your knuckles in a circular fashion. Exhale and repeat if necessary.

WEIGHT TRAINING AND STRETCHING.

Repeat Day 58 today. Remember that you always get the kind of development you want when you train specifically for it. If you want a full look to your muscles, then keep training with heavier weights. If you want a leaner, more defined look, then use the same weight, but cut down on the rest time between sets.

Day 73

AEROBIC EXERCISE

Before you begin your aerobic work today, sit in a quiet, comfortable place and mentally relax your body. Begin at your toes and work your way slowly up, breathing deeply, as you mentally, visually and physically relax completely. When you feel totally relaxed, remember your time for Jump Rope is 4 minutes and set your timer. Begin.

WEIGHT TRAINING AND STRETCHING

Repeat the Day-59 program. Increasing the intensity of your workout is fine and accelerates your progress when you feel good and your resistance is high; but if you are not feeling in top form, beware of overtraining. As time goes on you'll learn more and more how to understand the messages from your body. If you feel overtired it is better to rest than to force yourself to exercise. Don't be a compulsive exerciser, but at the same time don't use imagined weakness or fatigue as an excuse not to exercise. As you get to know your body better and better, you'll know what's best for you.

Day 74

AEROBIC EXERCISE

If you are someone who needs to lose weight and must constantly struggle to keep it under control, you've probably tried a low-calorie diet and found it very unsatisfying, leaving you feeling down and tired. How many pieces of celery can one eat anyway!? You've already found out that exercising is a better method of weight control than dieting. When you exercise you lose more fat than lean tissue. Usually on a fad diet (not the balanced type that we advocate) you lose more lean tissue than fat because you are almost constantly in a state of starvation. Your body must get nourishment from somewhere, so it gets some of it from the muscle. This is how, without exercise, you can lose size but still be fat and flabby. Did you know that just by walking briskly you can burn up around 350 calories an hour! And by jogging, 500 calories an hour? If you added either of these forms of exercise to your program, your progress would be hastened.

For Jump Rope today, set your timer for 4 minutes and 30 seconds.

WEIGHT TRAINING AND STRETCHING

Today, repeat the Day-57 program. The ideal way to develop a hard look to your body and to lose unwanted body fat is by resting only when your partner is doing his/her exercise and stretch. Exercising at this pace is very difficult and takes some adjusting to—and of course, you can't train as heavily with the weights. With this approach your muscles will not be as big, but they will become more defined.

Day 75

AEROBIC EXERCISE

Doing a variety of aerobic activities adds a lot of fun to your exercise regimen. Besides increasing your endurance and conditioning your heart and lungs, jumping rope can give you more coordination and improve your skills in sports of any kind. Today your aerobic time is 5 minutes.

WEIGHT TRAINING AND STRETCHING

Repeat the Day-58 program today. We tend to identify with the person who is our training partner to some extent—that is, we tend to achieve the same kind of results. This is great if your goals and your partner's goals are similar. If your goals are very different, however, you must make allowances for each other's individual programs. If you live with the person with whom you train, this tendency is even more obvious. We notice this in our own lives. When one gains weight so does the other, because we both tend to eat more.

Conversely, when Frank is training to get into competition condition, Christine gets into her best condition too. It is important to take advantage of each other's support but also to respect each other's individuality as well. This affinity develops with experience. Also, since people have different physical makeups, each exercise will affect each person differently; and the effect that one partner may feel intensely from an exercise, his/her partner may hardly feel at all. Concentrate on doing what feels best for you.

Day 76

AEROBIC EXERCISE

We haven't discussed the relationship of age to the amount or frequency of exercise. One reason is that we don't believe age has as much to do with your workout abilities as do your health and attitude toward exercising. We have seen people over 50 years old who are in better physical condition— with more pep, endurance and enthusiasm—than many youths we have come in contact with during our teaching years. If you pursue a vigorous way of life even at a mature age, you will continue to enjoy the health and rewards of being in shape. Your aerobic time for jumping rope today is 5 minutes and 30 seconds.

WEIGHT TRAINING AND STRETCHING

"Peaking" is the science of reaching a point of maximum physical condition by following a plan. We have found the ideal length for this plan to be 12 weeks. This is your last workout of your eleventh week. It is the Day-59 program. Now go and give it everything you've got!

Day 77

AEROBIC EXERCISE, WEIGHT TRAINING AND STRETCHING

You've made it almost all the way through your 3-month program! Get a good rest today. To really look your best, get a suntan. (See the section on tanning.) Sunning removes excess water from your body and makes your skin feel tighter. If it's the wrong time of the year for sunbathing, then consider taking a sauna, which also removes excess water from your system. Don't overdo it and be sure to drink a little extra water if you decide to relax in either of these ways.

MUTUAL-ASSISTANCE TECHNIQUE

Since you and your partner know you've already succeeded and accomplished your goals, reward your partner by taking him/her out to dinner. In this way you'll get to go out to dinner twice. At each dinner, offer a critique of each other's choice of food and beverage in a tactful and helpful way. Are these choices what they should be? Compliment your partner on the progress he/she has made concerning food selection.

BODY AWARENESS

Sitting in your private, comfortable place, close your eyes and mentally give yourself two positive suggestions about your present condition (referring to the progress of your attitude, diet or exercise as related to your body) and one positive suggestion for the future. This is something that you should begin working on very soon. On a clean page in your journal, write down any compliments you can give yourself about carrying out these suggestions. For example, you may say, "I have been very successful in following a healthful way of eating the past 11 weeks and shall continue to be successful." Compliment yourself by saying, "Congratulations (your name). You have done a magnificent job of following a healthful diet. I am very proud to be a part of you!" Do this for as many times as you can truthfully come up with a compliment. Now think of one negative aspect of yourself and then follow it with two more positive aspects. (If you can't think of any more, use what you just wrote in your journal.) Try to deal mainly with your diet, exercise, appearance or attitude. Now imagine someone whom you admire giving you a compliment about these positive aspects. Hear this person actually saying it in his/her own voice and speaking manner. Do this five times. Use different compliments as well as different people. Write down all the things that you experienced with regard to your body while doing this awareness exercise.

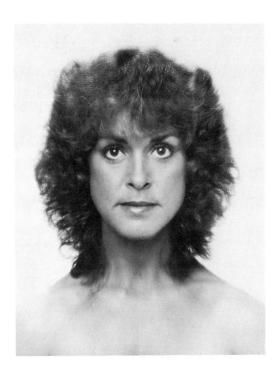

Week Twelve
Day 78

AEROBIC EXERCISE

Goals are very important. They are especially important in a physical fitness program like this. Today is the first day of the final week of this program. Take a look at the goals that you set for yourself to reach at the end of the 12-week program. Refresh your memory about exactly what you will be achieving by the eighty-fourth day. Visualize yourself already reaching this goal, and notice how quickly changes occur during these last few days. Be persistent and positive. Your aerobic time for Track Start is 3 minutes today.

WEIGHT TRAINING AND STRETCHING

You are really coming nearer to your goal and getting a lot of encouragement to meet it, which makes you feel wonderful. But it's not always that terrific. Sometimes when we are doing so well we meet up with someone who isn't doing quite as well, and he/she just can't bear having you feel good about yourself. He/she may make remarks about your wasting your time and even try to persuade you to "relax, have a good time, don't torture yourself." We've probably all heard remarks like this; and sometimes they cause us to work harder and other times they set us back. We don't allow things like this to effect us at all. Just remember, you are doing something of great value for yourself. You have developed a sense of accomplishment and your will has become stronger. Nothing can discourage you unless you allow it to. Don't let anything stand in your way to a great Day-57 workout today.

ADVANCED DIET TIP

Review the diet tips we have suggested during the past 11 weeks.

We feel it is of great value to continue keeping a good journal. You may want to personalize it as you expand it. Adding a section for nutritious recipes, or a section with names and addresses of restaurants you've enjoyed, rating and describing them briefly may be useful. Always reread your food records on a regular basis. This keeps you directed toward your goal. Share your discoveries with your partner and/or someone who shows interest in what you are doing. Never allow yourself to get discouraged. Instead of seeing things that occur as problems and defeats, see them as challenges and victories. A seemingly negative occurrence may turn out to be something positive for you in the long run.

Day 79

AEROBIC EXERCISE

Exercise stimulates your nervous system and your brain. You are probably noticing how much clearer your mind is and how much easier you seem to learn and remember things. Your blood gets an increase in oxygen and cleans out your entire system. This improvement in circulation is one of the wonderful benefits of exercise. When you are active you feel like doing more, having friends, and enjoying life to the utmost. If this were the only benefit you received from exercise, it would definitely still be worth it! Your aerobic time for Track Start is 3 minutes and 30 seconds.

WEIGHT TRAINING AND STRETCHING

Repeat the Day-58 workout for today. During this last week of your exercise program, relax as much as possible by closing your eyes and breathing deeply for intervals of a few minutes at a time throughout the day. We lose a big percentage of the energy available to us because we always have our eyes open and close them only when asleep. It is possible to get many of the beneficial effects of sleep by merely closing your eyes and relaxing. Sight is a dominant sense in most people, so conserve some of that energy by closing your eyes and relaxing periodically. Be sure, of course, to keep your eyes open during your workouts! Before and/or after your training is the best time to practice this form of relaxation.

Day 80

AEROBIC EXERCISE

We have given you a variety of aerobic exercises. These exercises give your heart and circulatory and respiratory systems a workout along with conditioning potential "problem" areas of your body. As you continue your program, feel free to add even more variety by trying a new sport. If you're presently cycling, try running for a few days. If you're a jogger, give skating a try. Adding variety makes your program more fun, time goes by more quickly and progress is faster.

Your aerobic time for Track Start is 4 minutes today. Remember, this is the minimum. Don't feel restricted to this time.

WEIGHT TRAINING AND STRETCHING

In a place where you can be alone and preferably facing a mirror, say aloud to yourself, "I create all doubts and negative attitudes about myself—no one else does this to me." Repeat this ten times or more.

Then repeat the following ten times: "I can create all positive feelings about myself. I am creating a super body!"

Judging from the progress you've made, it should be obvious to you how you've created your own body. Now go and re-create your body today with the Day-59 program.

Day 81

AEROBIC EXERCISE

You achieve both muscle endurance and muscle strength in this complete method of fitness. You gain muscle strength through the weight-training exercises and muscle endurance through the aerobic work and the repetitions. For example, in some of the weight exercises you are doing about 15 repetitions. In the aerobic work you may be doing over 100 repetitions. If you run, count your steps. Fifty repetitions is nothing! The advantages of muscle endurance come to view daily. Many of the activities you do each day —like typing, walking, digging, standing, etc.—are repetitive and require muscle endurance. When you increase your muscle endurance you decrease fatigue.

Your aerobic time for Track Start today is 4 minutes and 30 seconds.

WEIGHT TRAINING AND STRETCHING

When you're around people who exercise regularly and follow a good diet, you'll see in them a lot of energy and enthusiasm for life. They have a better outlook on what they are doing and on life in general. They don't become upset easily and can handle difficult situations better. They seem relaxed and confident in themselves. Does this sound like you? We know that the psychological benefits of the active life do exist for those who exercise regularly. Enjoy them! Repeat your Day-57 program.

Day 82

AEROBIC EXERCISE

As you exercise, notice the suppleness in your legs. Try Lunge on Step, without using any weight, as a warm-up exercise today. Follow this by the One-Leg-up Stretch. The time for Track Start today is 5 minutes.

WEIGHT TRAINING AND STRETCHING

We're sure you've met people who say they're too busy to exercise. Once we met a woman who made this claim but, in fact, she had servants who did everything from caring for her one child, cooking and cleaning, to gardening and odd jobs. All in all, she and her husband had about eight servants. She didn't have an outside job and didn't have to do anything at home. She and her husband owned a gym, which he, not she, was partially in charge of. She informed us that she didn't exercise. We asked her why, since it seemed she could devote all her time to this pursuit. She answered, "I have no time to exercise." Well she was overweight, so we knew she had some time . . . which she apparently spent overeating. She needed to reevaluate how she spent her time and see exactly what priority she placed upon·her health. We were visiting with her and her husband for a week, and by the time we left she was starting to realize the value of fitness. We didn't have to persuade her with verbal communication; we just did what we normally do—exercise and lead a healthful way of life. We've found that actions always speak louder than words.

Today repeat the program of Day 58.

Day 83

AEROBIC EXERCISE

This is your last aerobic workout of the entire program. You've come a long way and gotten into better shape as a result of doing these regularly. Your time for Track Start today is 5 minutes and 30 seconds. Do more if you want to!

WEIGHT TRAINING AND STRETCHING

Repeat the Day-59 program. You'll soon be finishing your 12-week program. You may want to use this book again to continue to give structure to your workouts. You'll find that each time you go through it you'll achieve more and more. If you feel you've learned enough to become independent, then use this book as a guide for planning your own personalized program and for future reference when you need a little incentive and guidance. When you first started out, you didn't know as much about your body as you do now. You've gained knowledge of which exercises and stretches work which areas, and you can now experiment and create your own successful program. Use the record you've kept for future reference. It will be invaluable.

Day 84

AEROBIC EXERCISE, WEIGHT TRAINING AND STRETCHING

After today, continue to step up your aerobic workouts by increasing your time gradually. Next week, for example, you may increase your beginning time to 3 minutes and 30 seconds as opposed to the present starting time of 3 minutes. Then each day increase in jumps of 30 seconds. This is enough to gain the benefits, but not too much to cause you to overdo the exercise. By following this gradual method of progression, your body will easily adjust and become accustomed to more and more aerobic work. Stay fit . . . Keep up . . . and don't quit!

You've really accomplished a great deal in the past 12 weeks. Think back to how it was during the first day of aerobics. Remember how long that minute felt? If you've kept a record throughout the 12 weeks, turn back to that first week and read your thoughts. Continue your progression forward. It may be time to set new goals and begin again.

MUTUAL-ASSISTANCE TECHNIQUE

Congratulations on successfully completing your program! Before you start again, take a few days off. Stay on a good diet during this layoff period and you'll notice the aftereffects of the exercise taking place. When you return to your exercise program, begin at a higher level on Day 1 of the Basic Program and go through it again. You may wish to train alone this time. This takes more discipline, especially if you've depended a great deal on the motivation of your partner.

We've trained both together and alone and have made progress both ways. If you get along well with your partner, then you'll probably enjoy training together again. If the individual differences between you and your partner are too great, you may want to choose another partner or train alone.

BODY AWARENESS

Today is the day you take your "after" photos. Be certain to take them under the very same conditions as before. Use the same equipment, and stand at the same distance from the camera. Take all views—front, right side, back, left side—in a relaxed pose, and have the photos developed in the same manner. Compare these shots with those taken previously. Where have you improved? Where do you still need to improve? Write down all the benefits of having made these changes. List as many as you can think of. Read them over when you're finished.

On a clean page of your journal's Body Awareness section, write down a plan of how you intend to carry on your fitness program for a lifetime of fitness. Be specific. Record all your feelings about your Body Awareness exercises.

ADVANCED PROGRAM	First Level			Middle Level			Top Level		
Day-57 Exercises	Weight Used	Sets	Reps	Weight Used	Sets	Reps	Weight Used	Sets	Reps
Hyperextension									
Forward Stretch									
Top Deadlift and Shrug									
Downward Neck Stretch									
Barbell Row									
One-Arm Lat Stretch— High									
Front or Behind- Neck Pulldown									
Sideways Swing									
One-Arm Dumbbell Row									
One-Arm Lat Stretch—Low									
Alternate Dumbbell Curl									
Push-ups, Fingers Back Stretch									
Dumbbell Incline Curl									
Arms-Backward Stretch with Pronation									
Dumbbell Concentration Curl									
Doorknob Isometric Curl									
Reverse Curl									
Fist Curl, Wrist Down									
Wrist Curl									
Wall Lean									
Incline Knee-in									
Bent-Leg Partial Sit-up									

ADVANCED PROGRAM	First Level			Middle Level			Top Level		
Day-58 Exercises	Weight Used	Sets	Reps	Weight Used	Sets	Reps	Weight Used	Sets	Reps
Push-ups (warm-up)									
Bench Press									
Doorway Stretch									
Incline Dumbbell Press									
Incline Stretch Between Chairs									
Decline Dumbbell Fly									
Pectoral Squeeze									
Dumbbell Pullover									
One-Arm Dumbbell Row									
Dip Stretch Between Chairs									
Dumbbell Press									
One-Arm Shoulder Stretch									
Barbell Front Raise									
Doorknob Isometric Front Raise									
Dumbbell Side Raise									
Doorway Isometric Lateral Stretch									
Dumbbell Rear Raise									
Doorway Isometric Front Stretch									
Close-Grip Bench Press									
Reverse Dip Stretch Between Chairs									
One-Arm Dumbbell Extension									
Overhead Stretch									
Dumbbell Kickback									
Arms-Backward Stretch									
Hanging Knee-up									
Seated Twist									

240

ADVANCED PROGRAM	First Level			Middle Level			Top Level		
Day-59 Exercises	Weight Used	Sets	Reps	Weight Used	Sets	Reps	Weight Used	Sets	Reps
One-Leg Top Extension (warm-up)									
Half Squat									
Lunge on Step									
One-Leg-up Stretch									
Leg Curl									
Stiff-Legged Deadlift									
Leg Extension									
Donkey Calf Raise									
Two-Leg Calf Stretch									
Standing Calf Raise									
Tibialis Toe Raise									
One-Leg Calf Raise									
Wall Lean (for calves)									
Hanging Knee-up									
Bent-Leg Partial Sit-up									
Seated Twist									

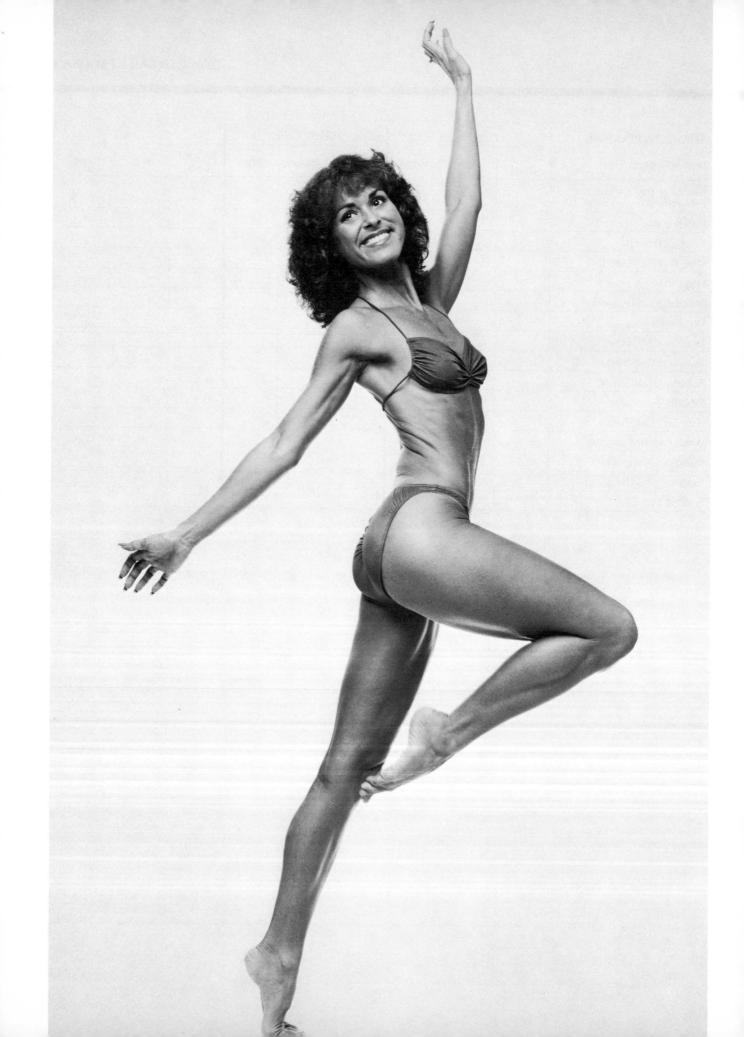

ENJOYING
YOUR BODY

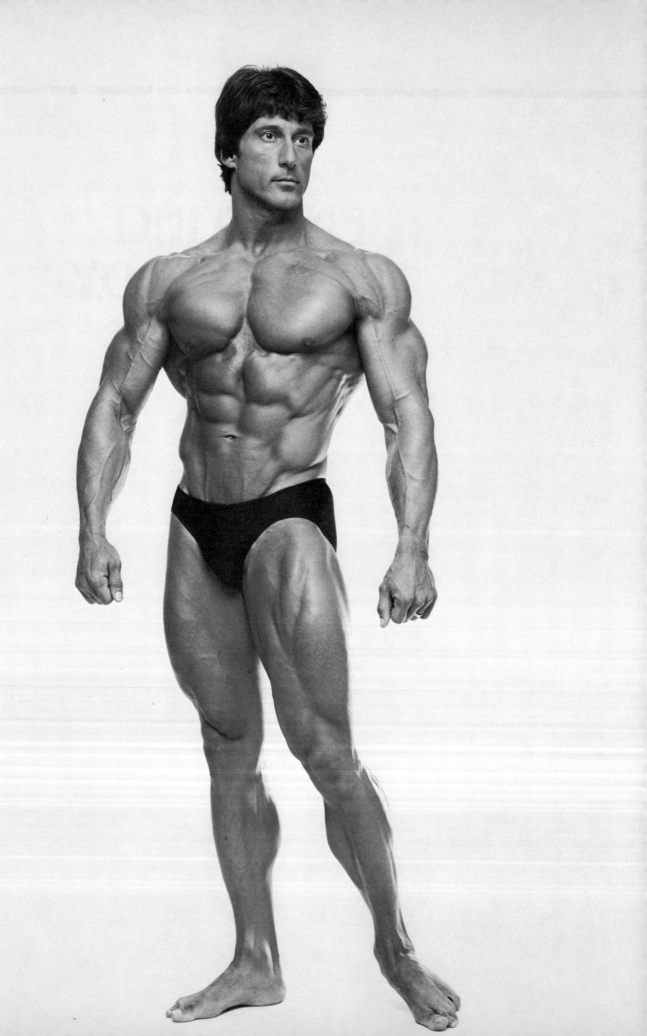

Sunning

When you are in shape and your energy is high, you enjoy your body to a greater degree. You can feel the sensual pleasures of life with greater intensity. It is as though the nerve endings were reaching out to seek pleasurable sensations. One of the easiest and most natural ways to give your body pleasure, and to nourish it at the same time, is by bathing in warm, soothing sunlight. Sunning not only provides you with essential Vitamin D, it gives your skin a tighter feel and firmer look. You will also have increased vitality as long as you don't stay in the sun too long and end up feeling drained. The secret of sunning is to do it gradually and not to stay out for prolonged periods. If you are lucky and possess an olive or dark complexion, you can handle the sun a little better than someone with fairer skin. Usually those with darker complexions have oilier skin, and the sun doesn't parch them so readily. But no matter what skin type you have, you should always take precautions. If you have oily skin use a lotion that is water based and has a sunscreen to filter out the burning rays. You will still get a tan, but you won't burn and turn red. If your skin is drier you can use an oil-based sunscreen. Don't use baby oil, which is essentially mineral oil. This is absorbed by the skin and may destroy some of the vitamins in your body. It can also block your pores and act as a cooking oil as well—literally frying you in the sun. This "cooking" effect happens with cocoa butter, too. Almond and sesame oil can be purchased at a health food store, and are very good for conditioning your skin while you sun. If you buy prepared sunning creams or oils, read the ingredients. Don't buy those with mineral oil. Stay with natural preparations. PABA and allantoin are ingredients to look for. PABA permits tanning while blocking the harmful burning rays. It is not a sun block but a sunscreen. Allantoin is a moisturizer that helps keep your skin soft and supple while sunning. It is also found in the herb comfrey; therefore drinking comfrey tea or making a paste out of powdered comfrey leaves and applying it to your skin after being in the sun can be helpful. Using these natural skin products can help you develop a long-lasting, evenly brown tan without harming your skin. If your skin is extremely sensitive, or you don't wish to get a tan, use an effective sun block, such as zinc oxide, which can be purchased as a lotion, gel or cream. Avoid too much sunning for your skin type and adjust your tanning to the type of climate you live in (remember you can get a burn when it's overcast too). Sunning during the intense sun hours from 11:00 A.M. to 2:00 P.M., using drugs (antibiotics, antihistamines) and eating certain foods (those with dyes or artificial sweeteners, for example) can cause bad reactions in some people. When you are sunning enjoy fresh, cool foods and clear mineral water.

For those who are unable to get a tan from the sun, there are always tanning lights and liquid tints and stains; however we don't recommend any of these. Tanning should be a pleasurable experience accompanied by the warmth of the sun, not poured from a bottle. Try to get a natural suntan no matter how little time you can spend working on it. It's like exercising—regularity is what counts.

After sunning use a good natural greaseless moisturizer on your skin. This should be applied as soon as you come out of a moderately warm to cool shower. Pat yourself dry, leaving a bit of moisture on your skin, and then apply the moisturizer—massaging it in well. If you are a bit damp the cream spreads more easily; and if you apply the moisturizer directly following a shower, your skin will absorb more. This will not only give you beautiful skin, but your tan will last longer.

Massage

Massage has existed for centuries as a form of medicine as well as pleasure. Proper circulation is essential for your well-being, and massage is an excellent way to work on specific areas of your body. It can also help stimulate your nerves, loosen tight joints and muscles and generally relax you. You don't need someone to give you a massage, though it is the most enjoyable and thorough way. You can do it yourself. The areas that tend to hold the most tension are within easy reach. When you massage your shoulder and neck area, do one side at a time. Use your left hand to massage your right shoulder and your right hand to massage your left shoulder. Gently knead these areas until you feel a warmth from increased circulation. With both hands, softly press with your fingertips in an alternating fashion, move into your neck area and then on to your scalp. With your fingertips rub and massage, thoroughly stimulating the blood flow in the scalp. Do this all over your head in a gentle, nonpulling way. Use some cream or moisturizer on your face for a facial massage. Foot massage can be done easily on bare feet wherever you are and is very satisfying. Knead, rub and gently press all over your feet and ankles until they are warm and relaxed. Always massage gently, never in a rough, fast fashion. For variety use techniques like light pressure, rubbing, kneading, tapping, vibrating and rubbing in a circular motion. If you say you will massage someone else in exchange for a massage yourself, someone will probably accept your offer. Everyone enjoys a nice soothing, relaxing massage.

What we have just described is a simple, easy massage that takes no training; however, there are other types that you might want to look into in greater detail.

Reflexology, sometimes called zone therapy, is a method of massage for bringing your body back into balance. There are reflexes in your feet that correspond with the various organs and parts of your body. They are laid out like a map. Tenderness in these areas indicates an imbalance in the corresponding organ or part of the body. Massaging gently with your hands, stimulates the area and sends blood to help heal the unbalanced part. The hands also have the same reflexes and can be worked on in the same manner. Massaging these reflexes for ten minutes a day can encourage a flow of energy throughout your body giving you a feeling of revitalization.

Shiatsu, or accupressure, is a Japanese finger-pressure massage. It deals with the same points found in acupuncture treatment. Applying pressure on specific points will stimulate the corresponding gland, organ or body part, thereby sending blood to the area, and promoting better health through circulation. This is a gentle massage that can be done at home without equipment. There are many books available on the subject.

There are also Rolfing, Touch for Health and Polarity Therapy, but these should only be done by a trained therapist.

When you are massaging yourself, or being massaged by someone, try using ice. Freeze some water in a paper or Styrofoam cup. Peel the cup down so you can still hold it comfortably and the ice is exposed about two inches. In a circular fashion, rub over the pressure points on your feet, hands or other parts of your body until the area is red and well numbed. This pulls the blood inward, and when the area begins to warm, blood rushes back and remains longer than if it had been massaged without ice. If you do this before you lie down to rest, or before going to bed at night, the area that you treated will feel well and relaxed when you get up. The circulation will be increased while you are resting. In fact, massaging your feet with ice or bathing them in ice water before going to bed can help promote restful sleep.

Baths

Water has many therapeutic properties. A warm bath, to which herbs and minerals have been added, can help relax and revitalize your system. If you have ever been swimming in the ocean you may have felt the healing effects on your skin from the minerals present in salt water. Of course salt isn't the only mineral in the water. By adding any of the following herbs and minerals to your bath water you can simulate this effect.

1. Epsom salts, seaweed, sulphur, sea salt and soda—help relieve muscle soreness, fatigue and poor circulation.
2. Chamomile—soothing and healing effect on your skin. You can use tea bags on your eyes for a very relaxing result.
3. Chervil—soothes pain and skin irritations.
4. Elder flowers—a mild astringent effect, good for skin irritations, softens your skin.
5. Fennel—helps soften the skin and works to prevent wrinkles. It can also be used as a compress on your eyes to soothe inflamed and watery eyes. If you live in an area of intense pollution this treatment would be quite useful.
6. Horsetail—good astringent and good for brittle nails. Especially effective on tired feet.
7. Lady's mantle—good for skin irritations.
8. Lemon balm—very soothing to skin. It cleanses and conditions.
9. Marigold—a skin conditioner. Soothes skin eruptions or small scrapes.
10. Mints—helps relieve pain—almost an anesthetic effect. Promotes a fresh, clear complexion. The aroma seeping up from the bath water helps open and clear your breathing passages.
11. Rose geranium leaves—give off an aromatic, spicy odor when put in hot water.
12. Rosemary—improves the quality of your hair and skin.
13. Goldenrod—said to help speed up the healing of small wounds.
14. Summer savory—very aromatic when included in your bath water.
15. Thyme or lemon thyme—has a sweet odor which is good as a deodorant and perfume.
16. Yarrow—very cleansing and beautifying.
17. Eucalyptus—the aroma opens and clears your breathing passages. It refreshes your skin in much the same way mint does.
18. Lime flowers—smooths wrinkles and improves circulation.
19. Valerian—helps you get a more relaxed night's sleep.

These herbs can be used in combinations directly in your bath water, or as steams, compresses or pastes applied to specific areas. Many can be taken internally in the form of tea.

When bathing remember these principles: Warm water is generally used to relax and relieve tensions. It is also the best temperature for using herbs to aid skin ailments. The warm bath should be around 90 to 95 degrees Fahrenheit and can be soaked in for as long as it is comfortable. Hot baths begin at 100 degrees and open the skin's pores, allowing you to absorb easily the herbs in your bath. Heat draws the blood to the skin surface and you begin to sweat faster than in a warm bath; thus your skin is cleansed, muscle soreness and tiredness are released and your circulation is increased. A hot bath is very exhausting and should only be taken for short periods. You should have time to lie down, covered and away from drafts, to rest afterward. Cold baths are usually less than 60 degrees Fahrenheit and not taken for longer than two minutes. The cold water drives the blood away from the surface of the body and creates a longer-lasting warmth as the blood works its way back to all the blood vessels. Cold baths are very healing and energizing. Alternating hot with cold baths works like a pump to stimulate your blood flow. Stay in each bath no longer than 2 minutes and alternate about three times. Always end with the cold bath. If you have a difficult time in a cold bath, use a shower to splash cold water and warm to hot water on yourself. Always have a seat handy with slip-resistant legs in case you wish to sit down. Of course, children, the elderly, and those with heart trouble, anemia, nervous tension and other health problems should not take these baths.

One of our favorite baths is the hydro-massage. From powerful jets, hot water is forced out at a rapid rate creating a forceful massage. It is very stimulating to sore, fatigued muscles and releases stored tension. A whirlpool bath is similar but uses warm water and is not quite as forceful. But the swirling waters are very relaxing and helpful if you have a difficult time sleeping. Aerated baths are even gentler. They are created by air bubbles forced through small holes. Often hydro-massage contains aerated water as well.

Sitz baths can be either hot or cold and are generally for problems in the lower abdomen—intestines, genitals and so forth. Sit in water covering your lower body with your knees slightly elevated and, if desired, covered with a blanket to induce sweating. This is very calming and relaxing.

Steam bath temperatures range from 100 to 150 degrees Fahrenheit, and are created by pouring water over hot rocks or coals. Anywhere from 15 to 30 minutes is usually sufficient depending on the temperature. If the room is very hot or you're not accustomed to taking steam baths stay a little less time—possibly 5 minutes to begin with. You may feel a little dizzy from the loss of fluid, but this generally happens after you leave the bath. Use a brush or loofah sponge while sweating heavily to cleanse and brush away all dead skin. Follow this with a cold shower to draw the blood inward and close the pores. Don't wait until you feel dizzy or your heart begins to beat quickly to leave the bath. Leave and reenter as often as you feel necessary. To protect the top of your head while in the steam room, wrap it with a cool, moist, natural-fiber cloth.

Sauna baths are very similar to steam except they use dry heat.

Coals or rocks are heated to temperatures of 190 to 200 degrees Fahrenheit, but no water is used. This type of bath is good for drying up the sinuses and relaxing tired, sore muscles. Stay in the sauna for short periods of time—no more than 15 minutes, and less if you are a beginner. Follow the sauna with a cold shower as you did with the steam bath. Always protect your head with a cool, natural-fiber cloth.

Enjoy all the various types of baths. Use them for healing purposes or for pleasure. You will feel much better, and your skin will acquire a healthy glow. Massage yourself, or better yet, get a massage immediately afterward. This is the optimum time because your muscles are relaxed and more easily manipulated. After a short rest, you will feel completely renewed.

Sleep

Sleep is one of the most important aspects of your program. Without it, repairs can't take place and you feel tired and irritable. When you first begin exercising you may feel overtired and exhausted. This feeling will not last very long. It is caused by the toxicity of your system, and through exercise and proper diet this will soon be eliminated. Take naps to help combat the fatigue in the meantime. When you sleep, wear as little clothing as possible or sleep in very loose, natural-fiber clothing; in a dark, well-ventilated room with fresh air circulating freely. If you have plants in your bedroom remove them at night. This is the time when they give off carbon dioxide. During the day they give off oxygen. Go to bed before midnight, and you will find that you will get more restful and deeper sleep. If you have a difficult time falling asleep, take a warm mineral/herb bath and drink some valerian or chamomile tea. Also taking the amino acid L-Tryptophan helps induce a deep sleep without a "drug" effect. Spend some time meditating, breathing deeply and consciously relaxing your body.

When you get up in the morning do so in a slow, relaxed manner. Never jump out of bed and begin rushing madly about. First stretch and yawn, then turn and twist slowly until you feel awake. Next, sit up and continue stretching and yawning while still in bed. Stand up slowly and stretch some more. Drink some water that is at room temperature with a little squeeze of fresh lemon in it. It will help your system to begin working and encourage elimination of food left in your intestines. Now dress warmly in loose clothing and prepare yourself for your aerobic work.

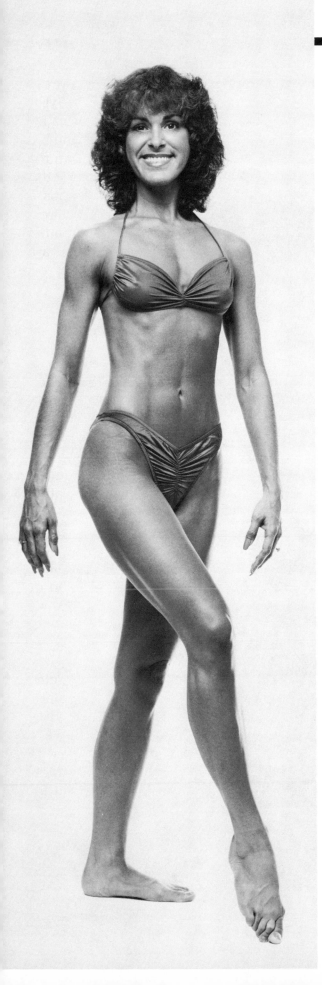

USEFUL INFORMATION

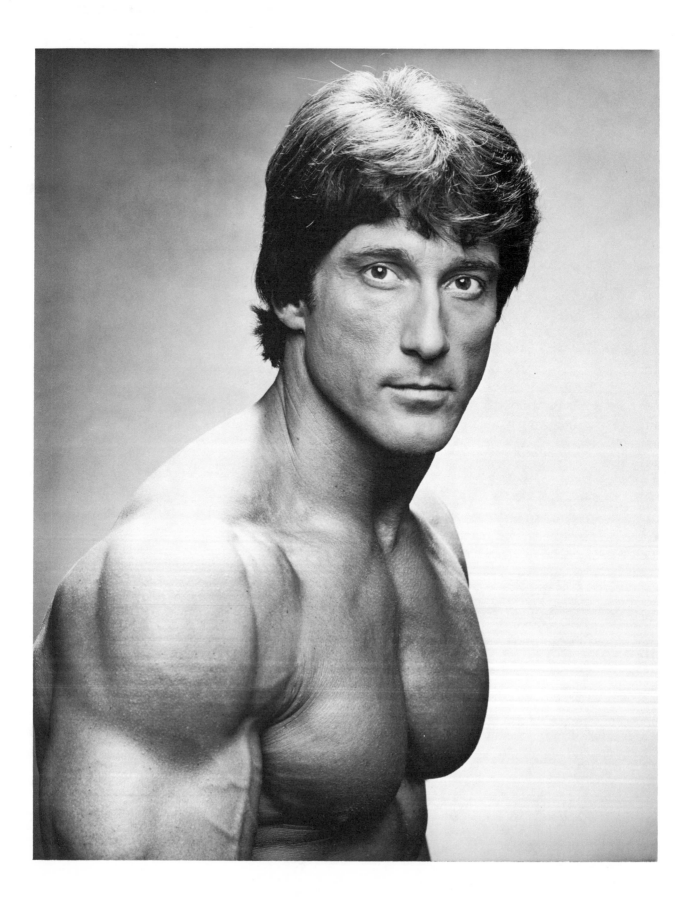

Interrupting Your Training

"What happens when you stop training?" is a question we are frequently asked. Sometimes it is necessary to stop for a while. If you are feeling very tired and sore, you may be overtraining. Take a one- to three-day break and then resume normal training at the point where you left off. Or if you are forced to take a few weeks off because of work or family obligations, then start back on an easier program. If you take more than one week off before you finish the Basic Program then, start again at Day 1. If you take more than one week off before you finish the Intermediate Program, start back at Day 29. If you take more than one week off before you finish the Advanced Program, start back at Day 57. The longer you stop training the more you will tend to return to the condition you were in before you started. Frank tends to lose weight when he stops, but Christine gains weight. Muscles do not and cannot turn to fat, because they are a different type of tissue. If you stop exercising but keep eating the same amount as when you were exercising, you may gain weight because the extra calories and carbohydrates are not burned up.

Self-Motivation

Getting in shape requires discipline. We know that we both get into better shape when we have a special event for which we must look our best. Self-motivation is really a matter of personal responsibility. You must decide what is more important to you: achieving your goal by closely following your training and nutritional program—or the temporary pleasure that comes from breaking your training or going off your diet. Not only are you responsible for this choice, but since your own self-motivation and behavior influence your partner's attitude, you are also partially responsible for his/her attitude as well. Thinking this way will help keep you motivated.

Problem Areas—Building and Reducing

There may be certain parts of your body that aren't responding the way you would like. These "stubborn body parts" need more work than the more responsive areas. Below are listed exercise sequences that will quickly shape up any lagging body parts. Do the exercises in the order listed twice a week in addition to your regular workout. Do them on the days when you don't train that body part. Use the same number of sets and reps that you are currently using in the program, or do the sets and reps as listed. You should notice an improvement within two or three weeks. These extra routines shock or surprise the body and force it to respond. Don't do them for more than two or three weeks at a time because after this your body adjusts to them. Use a weight that allows you to do the suggested repetitions.

	BUILD	REDUCE
CALVES		
Donkey Calf Raise	5 sets, 15 reps	3 sets, 30 reps
Two-Leg Calf Stretch	5 sets, 20 sec	3 sets, 20 sec
One-Leg Calf Raise	5 sets, 15 reps	3 sets, 15 reps
One-Leg Calf Stretch	5 sets, 20 sec	3 sets, 20 sec
THIGHS		
	Do only 1 additional time per week	
One-Leg Top Extension	4 sets, 15 reps	
Half Squat	4 sets, 8 reps	
Hack Squat	4 sets, 8 reps	
Stiff-Legged Deadlift	4 sets, 10 reps	
Leg Extension		4 sets, 25 reps
Lunge on Step		4 sets, 15 reps
Forward Stretch		4 sets, 20 sec
Leg Curl		4 sets, 15 reps
HIPS		
Lunge on Step		4 sets, 15 reps
Stiff-Legged Deadlift		4 sets, 15 reps
Half Squat		4 sets, 25 reps,
Hyperextension		4 sets, 20 reps
Seated Twist		100 reps
WAIST		
Hanging Knee-up		4 sets, 25 reps
Bent-Leg Partial Sit-up		4 sets, 25 reps
Incline Knee-in		4 sets, 25 reps
Seated Twist		100 reps
BACK		
Pulldown, Wide-Grip Chin or Letdown	4 sets, 8 reps	4 sets, 12 reps
Barbell Row	4 sets, 8 reps	4 sets, 15 reps
Top Deadlift and Shrug	4 sets, 8 reps	4 sets, 15 reps
Dumbbell Row	4 sets, 8 reps	4 sets, 12 reps
Hyperextension	4 sets, 12 reps	4 sets, 20 reps

CHEST

Bench Press	4 sets, 8 reps	4 sets, 15 reps
Incline Dumbbell Press	4 sets, 8 reps	4 sets, 12 reps
Dumbbell Fly	4 sets, 8 reps	4 sets, 15 reps
Dumbbell Pullover	4 sets, 8 reps	4 sets, 12 reps

SHOULDERS

Dumbbell Press	4 sets, 8 reps	4 sets, 15 reps
Barbell Front Raise	4 sets, 8 reps	4 sets, 15 reps
Dumbbell Side Raise	4 sets, 8 reps	4 sets, 15 reps
Dumbbell Rear Raise	4 sets, 8 reps	4 sets, 15 reps

TRICEPS

Dumbbell Kickback	3 sets, 8 reps	3 sets, 15 reps
Close-Grip Bench Press	3 sets, 8 reps	3 sets, 15 reps
Two-Arm Dumbbell Extension	3 sets, 8 reps	3 sets, 15 reps

BICEPS

Alternate Dumbbell Curl	3 sets, 8 reps	3 sets, 15 reps
Dumbbell Incline Curl	3 sets, 8 reps	3 sets, 15 reps
Dumbbell Concentration Curl	3 sets, 8 reps	3 sets, 15 reps

FOREARMS AND WRISTS

Reverse Curl	3 sets, 12 reps	3 sets, 20 reps
Wrist Curl	3 sets, 12 reps	3 sets, 20 reps

How to Get Stronger by Using Negative Resistance and Forced Repetitions

Negative resistance is an ideal way to build strength as well as muscle size. Take a count of 7 seconds to complete each repetition: Raise the weight up for 2 seconds, hold at peak muscle contraction for 1 second, and lower slowly for a count of 4 seconds. This uses negative resistance. You lower the weight twice as slowly as you raise it since you are physiologically 40 percent stronger on the negative or eccentric part of the exercise. Negative resistance is most effective for strength and size gains when 6 to 8 repetitions are used.

Forced repetitions enable you to get more out of each set by having your partner actually take weight off the bar, or lessen the weight with two fingers under the bar. This is done when you can't do any more reps on your own, so your partner helps you to do 2 or 3 additional reps, thereby working the muscle more deeply. Forced reps should only be done on your last set of exercises for all muscle groups except abdominals.

Using forced reps and/or negative resistance may cause deep muscular soreness and shouldn't be practiced all the time. These techniques should only be used on one exercise per body part (only competitive bodybuilders would use forced reps on every exercise and then only in their last 4 to 6 months before a competition). Be sure to warm up very thoroughly with lighter weights before using either of these methods.

How to Gain 10 Pounds of Solid Body Weight

It is possible to gain 10 pounds of relatively solid weight in 4 to 8 weeks. This added body weight will not be all muscle because any time you "bulk up" or gain weight quickly, some of it will be fat. A good plan is to gain 10 pounds and then cut back 5 pounds by lowering your daily calorie and carbohydrate intake. To stimulate muscular growth and gain, the bigger muscle groups should be concentrated on. Do this program three times a week for 8 weeks. Increase weight by 10 pounds each set on barbell and 5 pounds on dumbbell exercises each week because stronger muscles mean bigger muscles.

Half Squat—5 sets, 8 reps
Lunge on Step—3 sets, 8 reps
Donkey Calf Raise—5 sets, 15 reps
Bench Press—5 sets, 8 reps
Incline Dumbbell Press—3 sets, 8 reps
Press Behind Neck—3 sets, 8 reps
Top Deadlift and Shrug—5 sets, 8 reps
Barbell Row—3 sets, 8 reps
Alternate Dumbbell Curl—3 sets, 8 reps
Hanging Knee-up—4 sets, 25 reps

Rest as much as possible on the days when you don't train. You will need to eat more too. A nutritionist friend of ours has had great success with his students by having them take 6 raw egg yolks daily in light beer. Here's how: Fill a tall thin glass with 2 ounces light beer, drop in 2 egg yolks and drink it down. You won't even taste the egg yolks (make sure the yolks are whole). Do this three times daily. Also eat more dairy products like milk, yogurt and cheese (cottage cheese is especially good). Meats, whole-grain bread, fresh fruit and vegetables should make up the rest of your diet. Also add one or two small protein drinks daily (such as the ones we describe) made with milk-egg protein powder. In general, increase your calorie consumption, especially those calories that come from increased protein intake. More protein will give you more solid muscle weight gains.

How to Lose 10 Pounds Quickly in a Healthy Manner

Many of us have found ourselves in the situation where we have put on an extra 5 or 10 pounds and hadn't even realized it. It's as though we woke up and there it was—10 pounds more registering on our scale! The first thing we recommend is immediately begin to write down everything you eat and keep track of the calories, carbohydrates and grams of protein. This will help get you back on the right path to a healthier, slimmer body and will really open your eyes to what put on that extra weight. After a day of writing down your foods in a journal, read over what you have eaten. First look at the types of foods that you are eating. Are you getting a great deal of foods that contain empty calories, as we discussed earlier in the book? If so, this is where you should be cutting back—or preferably cutting them out completely. Do you eat more helpings than you should at meals? Cutting down on your portions will also help you to get back in shape quickly. Do you eat late at night? We suggest not eating after 7:00 P.M. because you will not be doing enough exercise to burn off the foods you eat after this time. In fact your evening meal should be very light. Be sure to get enough protein in your diet to satisfy and nourish the body. Generally if you want to lose a pound you must consume 3,500 fewer calories. If you stay on a diet high in protein and low in carbohydrates, this situation changes. You can eat more calories and still lose fat. The drop in weight takes place because the protein is used to feed your muscles, and with little carbohydrate being ingested your body begins to burn the fat that you have stored for energy purposes. When you are eating a diet that is higher in carbohydrates, your body uses the carbohydrates taken in as energy, making it necessary for you to exercise more to burn off the excess you have stored. We aren't saying to avoid all carbohydrates. We all need carbohydrates so that our brain and organs will function properly. We are saying: Choose your carbohydrates more carefully. Get full nutrition from what you eat. If you feel you need fruit in your diet, choose half a cantaloupe weighing about 1 pound, which has 68 calories and 17 grams of carbohydrate, instead of having the same amount of grapes (1 pound), which has 270 calories and 70 grams of carbohydrate! Quite a difference when you want to lose 10 pounds fast.

We suggest that you begin the day with a protein-rich breakfast. Have ⅛ wedge of a medium cantaloupe or 6 ounces of fresh watermelon. Eat two eggs fixed any style you wish as long as there is nothing added. With your eggs have ½ cup cottage cheese (low-fat) or a 1-ounce slice of mozzarella cheese. You may have a half slice of whole-grain bread, lightly buttered, if you wish. Have an herb tea for your beverage. This should fill you and satisfy your needs for all the food groups. Do not snack between meals unless it is only a bit of a protein food that contains no carbohydrates. Your lunch should come about 3½ to 4 hours after finishing your breakfast and should consist of ½ cup of tuna or chicken salad (prepared with 1 teaspoon of mayonnaise), or a 3- to 4-ounce serving of fresh broiled fish (sea bass, red snapper and unbreaded sole are very low in calories and high in protein), or one piece of broiled chicken (white meat has a lot fewer calories than dark meat), or ¼ of a medium avocado sprinkled with a little chili powder. If you are having a salad you can mix the avocado in it, but we feel it is better eaten alone. It will give you the feeling that you are having more to eat. Complement your lunch with a cool mixed green salad (1 cup). Use a variety of lettuce and add a mushroom and some alfalfa sprouts, and spice it with pepper, paprika and a little celery seed. Have a cool glass of mint tea with your meal.

For dinner eat a medium-sized salad which contains a variety of low-calorie and low-carbohydrate vegetables. Butter lettuce, red leaf lettuce, iceberg lettuce and watercress make a very tasty base. Add to this mixture any of the following: grated zucchini, yellow crooked-neck squash, sliced celery, grated eggplant, sliced radish, chopped onion, (try red onions, they are very sweet), alfalfa sprouts or fresh, steamed, cold asparagus. Use a vinegar and peanut oil dressing (no more than 2 teaspoons oil) with a little dry mustard and paprika mixed in, over the salad. Finish the meal with a cup of chamomile tea with a very thin slice of lemon floating in the cup. If you absolutely must have a late snack it should only be sparkling mineral water or a 6-ounce glass of chilled tomato juice or vegetable mix (like V-8). A good way to extend the juice is to add a few ice cubes and blend it well in the blender, a dash of celery seed while blending will give it a nice taste.

Dieting is the best way to reduce pounds quickly. To hasten the process and keep your body toned and fit you should also get more exercise. Do more for the areas that need it most. If you hold weight in your waist, do more Knee-ins and Twists. If your thighs need shaping up, do more walking, jogging, leg lunges and High Kicks. Of course the most important thing to remember is to keep your attitude positive. Look through the book and do some of the Body Awareness exercises in the Intermediate and Advanced sections. These exercises are designed to keep you moving toward your goal. With the diet we have outlined above, the increase in exercising and your ever-positive attitude, your 10 pounds will be gone very quickly.

Pregnancy and Exercising

Frank and I do not have children of our own, but we are godparents to a very beautiful young lady named Cherí and have shared in her life since she was first conceived. Both of our families have children. My sisters, all three of them, have a combined total of seven children, and Frank's brother has just become the father of his first child, Adam F. Zane. So our experience with pregnancy is more indirect than direct.

If you have been exercising regularly before pregnancy, you will find you have an easier time giving birth and your recovery will be much faster. Your back and abdominal muscles will be stronger and better able to carry this new weight around. Your overall health will be better, and your heart and circulatory systems will be in excellent condition to take any extra stress. You should, of course, consult your doctor before continuing your exercise program. Everything you do during pregnancy affects your child directly or indirectly. You need exercise, but you shouldn't strain or overwork yourself. Don't jump into a program that you've never done before. After the third month, do less and less strenuous exercising. For example, in your aerobics don't run or jog, instead do more up-tempo walking.

During pregnancy and childbirth there are some muscles you use more than others. Therefore, these should be strengthened to assist you at the right time. Involuntary muscles are aided by exercise just as voluntary muscles are. Your circulation, elimination, and heart work much better and easier as a result of exercise. The abdominal muscles are voluntary muscles and should be able to contract and relax at will for the force you will need to give birth to your child. The muscles in the lower pelvic area around the vagina must be able to be controlled so they can relax and allow the baby's head to pass easily. These muscles aren't generally used except in childbirth so you should learn to isolate them. Your back muscles are very important. Since you are carrying this added weight in the front of you, your back tries to compensate and reestablish balance. If your back isn't strong and in good shape, you could get backaches and stiffness. Keep this area loosened up and exercised. Your diaphragm must be in good condition for all the breathing and forcing you will be doing. In the exercise and stretching sections of this book you will find exercises to help strengthen this area; however, there are some precautions you should take. Use your arms to assist you if you do Sit-ups, and make sure that your knees are always bent. Don't strain the abdomen. When you do forward-stretching or upward-stretching movements, do them slowly and carefully. They are very good for keeping your back loose and in shape. Don't lie on your stomach. You don't want to place any unnecessary pressure on your abdomen. If you practice yoga, stay away from inverted postures such as head and shoulder stands. Don't do the stomach vacuum exercise: This causes an unnecessary pushing of the abdomen. Sitting cross-legged and in a squatting position helps to tone the muscles needed in childbirth. Exercise in well-ventilated rooms and use common sense. Move slowly and don't attempt any movements that you don't have complete control of.

Your diet should be perfect before childbirth and after. Remember, anything that enters your system also affects your child's system. Would you want your child taking drugs, alcohol, smoking cigarettes or developing a sweet tooth and an addiction to caffeine before birth? (Cola, coffee and chocolate contain caffeine.)

Exercising after giving birth is as important as before. It can give you a lot of energy, shape up your body and aid in preventing a great many problems that can result from giving birth. You will help your body regain its former condition and improve your circulation, so that your body can be fed the nourishment that it so desperately needs at this time. Start your exercise program as a beginner, staying away from anything strenuous. If you have been on a good diet before and during your pregnancy, you shouldn't have any problems with stretch marks or being overweight. If you do find yourself with some unwanted pounds, shed them gradually. Begin following your healthful way of eating, and before long you will see yourself shaping up. Get plenty of high-nutrition foods including high-quality protein and complex carbohydrates. Don't eliminate dairy products. You need them for calcium and protein and for your skin. Stick to a diet that is cleansing, full of fresh fruits and vegetables. Your skin and attitude will glow from it. Be patient with yourself. You need all the strength that you can summon to care for your child and for yourself. Feel happy and energetic with your new baby.

How to Exercise When Traveling

When you are on the road and have little time for exercise, try this routine which uses no equipment and can be done in your hotel room:

Track Start—1 to 3 minutes
Push-ups—10 to 20 reps
Doorway Isometric Lateral Stretch—hold 10 seconds
Doorway Isometric Front Stretch—hold 10 seconds
One-Arm Lat Stretch—hold 10 seconds each arm
Pectoral Squeeze—hold 10 seconds
Dip Stretch Between Chairs—hold 10 seconds
Doorknob Isometric Curl—hold 10 seconds

Lunge on Step—10 to 20 reps each leg
Free-Standing Calf Raise (on step)—25 reps
One-Leg-up Stretch—hold 10 seconds each leg
Flat Bench Knee-in—20 to 30 reps
Seated Twist—50 reps

Do this program every day if possible. It will get your circulation going and revitalize you!

Fitness in 10 Minutes a Day When Time Is Limited

If you're on a tight schedule and pressed for time but still want to stay in shape, you can remain in reasonably good condition in 10 minutes a day. It is very important to move from one exercise to the next with as little rest as possible between sets. Don't try to use heavy weights, but concentrate on doing each movement correctly. You will work upper body one day and lower body the next day.

Upper Body

Jump Rope—1 minute total
Bench Press—1 set of 15 reps
Overhead Stretch—hold 10 seconds
Press Behind Neck—1 set of 15 reps
Barbell Row—1 set of 15 reps
Two-Arm Dumbbell Extension—1 set of 15 reps
Barbell Curl—1 set of 12 reps
Reverse Curl—1 set of 12 reps
Flat Bench Knee-in—1 set of as many reps as possible

Lower Body

Jump Rope—1 minute total
One-Leg Top Extension—1 set of 15 reps each leg
Half Squat—1 set of 15 reps
Lunge on Step—1 set of 15 reps
Stiff-Legged Deadlift—1 set of 10 reps
One-Leg Calf Raise—1 set of 15 reps each leg
Free-Standing Calf Raise—1 set of 25 reps
Hanging Knee-up—1 set of 25 reps
Seated Twist—1 set of 50 reps

Do this program 6 days a week and rest on the seventh day.

Lifetime Maintenance Program

Your program for a Super Body in 12 Weeks can be used as a lifetime exercise program. To make continuous progress, follow the program at the first level the first time through, then take a week off and resume training at the middle level, Day 1, and go through the 12-week program again. Then another week off and begin the program again at Day 1 but at the top level. You will get into your best shape after you complete the top level. Then another week off and begin at middle level, Day 1. This will take you through a full year of training. Each time you go through the program, you will be stronger and able to use heavier weights and/or more repetitions. Adjust your poundages according to your goal, remembering that heavy weights and low reps build muscle size and strength, while high reps and less weight develop leaner, more defined muscle.

You can also stay at the same level each time you go through the 12-week program, just adjust your weights accordingly. First or middle level are the best programs to stay on for maintenance. Choose whatever level feels best to you.

Exercising for Sports

The table that follows is a guide to which exercises to do for thirteen different sports. If you wish to get stronger and improve your condition for a specific sport, do the exercises in the column under your sport in the order indicated by the numbers. Practice this program three times a week (twice a week during the season for your sport). Each program works the entire body but emphasizes those muscles most involved in the sport at hand. Start with 2 sets of 10 repetitions on upper-body exercises and 2 sets of 15 repetitions for lower-body work. Do 25 reps on waist exercises. After 3 weeks go to 3 sets of 10 on upper body, 3 sets of 15 on lower body and 3 sets of 30 on waist.

Injuries

Injuries are very common in any athletic activity, but many can be prevented through common sense. If you don't take the time to warm up properly and loosen your muscles until they are flexible, you could pull a muscle. If you are not nourishing your body well you may get injuries due to vitamin and mineral depletions. If your muscles are not in shape to handle the program you choose to do, you could suffer an injury. If you try to start an exercise program without beginning slowly and gradually increasing the amount you do (as we suggest in this 12-week program), or if you try to do too much at once

EXERCISES: / SPORTS	BOWLING	ARCHERY	CYCLING	HORSEBACK RIDING	VOLLEYBALL	BASKETBALL	SKATING	RUNNING	BASEBALL	FOOTBALL	GOLF	TENNIS	SWIMMING
Front Raise	3	2		9			8	7	9	15	4	9	5
Seated Twist	16	18	17	15	18	17	19	16	21			19	
Wide-Grip Chin or Letdown	1	3	6	12	3	8			6	11	2	6	2
Sideways Swing					4				7	12	3	7	3
Alternate Dumbbell Curl		10					13						
Wrist Curl		12							19		13	19	
Incline Knee-in	15	17		16					20	21	18	20	
Dumbbell Fly	2		10				6	6	8		9	8	4
Dumbbell Press			5		8	9	7			10	1		1
Dumbbell Side Raise	5	4	7	10	9	10	9	8	10	16	5	10	6
Dumbbell Rear Raise	8	5	8	11	10	11	10	9	11	17	6	11	7
Two-Arm Dumbbell Extension		12			11								10
Stiff-Legged Deadlift			14	5			4			4			
Bench Press					1	6				7			
One-Leg Top Extension			1	2		1	1	1	1	1		1	14
Dumbbell Pullover					5			14	14			14	9
Half Squat			2	3	14	2	2	2	2	2		2	15
One-Arm Shoulder Stretch	4	6							16		10	15	8
Barbell Row				4		12				13			
One-Arm Lat Stretch	7	9	12		7	14	12	11	13	14	8	13	12
Donkey Calf Raise	14	16	4	1	16	5	5	5	4	6	16	5	18
Barbell Curl	10			13	12	15							
Reverse Curl	11	14	13	14	13	16	14	13	17	20	13	18	
Hyperextension	13		15	6		4	17	4		5	17	4	17
Top Deadlift and Shrug		7	8	7			16			7			
One-Arm Dumbbell Row	6	8	11		6	13	11	10	12		7	12	11
Incline Dumbbell Press		1			2	7			5	8			
Dumbbell Kickback	9	11	9				15	15	15	18	11	16	
Hanging Knee-up			16		17	18	18	17					
Lunge on Step	12	15	3	4	15	3	3	3	3	3	13	3	16

and overtrain yourself, you can get injured. All of these things set you back. Usually when you are injured it is a result of trying to save time in your workouts. Hurrying doesn't save time—it costs you time!

If you are injured, first and foremost consult your doctor (preferably one acquainted with sports medicine) to determine what type of injury you have and how bad it is. Most injuries are minor and can be taken care of at home. We have found that the best thing to do as soon as you even slightly suspect an injury is to rest and apply an ice pack to the injured area. This will take the swelling down and help alleviate the pain. Heat is not used because it isn't always the best way to treat all injuries and can cause swelling to increase rather than decrease. Use ice first. One injury we all seem to develop is soreness in the muscles. This discomfort often takes anywhere from 12 to 48 hours to develop, depending on the nature of your activity. If you are sore from exercising, don't stop; instead exercise at a slower pace; use lighter weights and do higher repetitions. This will help work out the soreness and create circulation of blood in the area to promote healing. Soreness is normal. It usually is a sign that you are using muscles that you haven't used lately, or that you are building new tissue and capillaries. If you warm up properly you won't get as sore. If you are chronically sore you should consult your doctor and rest. You are probably overtraining and need to take it easy.

If you pull or tear a muscle, the best thing to do is exercise the area very, very lightly to get the blood circulating. Give it a great deal of rest and apply ice packs. When you start to exercise again, begin your program as a beginner for this area, and work on building up strength in the muscle so that it will not be as susceptible to injury again.

Another common injury is the muscle cramp or spasm, which is a sudden and lasting contraction of a muscle. This condition is very painful and can be felt in many degrees from a slight twinge to a full, hard, intense contraction. Cramps can be caused, for example, by not warming up properly, a strain of the muscle or blood not getting to the muscle. If your diet is low in vitamins and minerals (especially calcium, magnesium, potassium, Vitamins E and B_6) you are also susceptible to cramps. If cramping is a problem for you, we suggest adding more vitamins and minerals to your diet and warming up thoroughly before you exercise.

Tendinitis is an inflamed tendon which swells up and is very painful. When the tendon is exercised it stops hurting and the swelling goes down, but when you are finished exercising it reoccurs. This can persist for a long time. If tendinitis is a problem for you, exercise very slowly and with less strain on the area. Doing more stretching movements can also be helpful.

Lower-back pain is a common problem. It can be caused by stretching the ligaments too much in that area or by your back being out of alignment. A good chiropractor can help readjust your back and alleviate the pain. Do exercises that help strengthen the abdominal muscles (such as Bent-Leg Partial Sit-ups or Knee-ins) and build up the lower back (such as Forward Stretches). Do these exercises very carefully and gradually build up the number of repetitions. You will experience a little soreness, but this will be an indication that you are working the muscles. Don't overdo. When doing any exercise that requires you to bend over, always bend your knees to take the stress off your lower back. Never pick up objects from the floor without bending your knees and using your legs for assistance. Never do Sit-ups with your legs straight; always bend your knees. Never step into a car one foot at a time; sit on the seat first.

To protect yourself against knee injuries you should do exercises that strengthen them. Leg extensions are excellent for this purpose. This exercise is explained on page 209 using a machine. It can also be done without a machine by using weighted iron boots or ankle weights and sitting on the end of a table or high chair.

Preventing injuries through proper warming up and through strengthening the area with the proper exercise movements is the best way to stay healthy, avoid injuries and continually improve and get into top shape. Always be sure that you are wearing the proper shoes and training gear. Train in a gradual manner and don't allow yourself to become overtrained. Whenever you add a new movement to your program, start doing it as though you are a beginner—no matter how advanced you are. Don't neglect your stretching movements. Staying flexible is one way to prevent a great many injuries. When you exercise, aim for a balanced development. If you are doing a sport that can cause an imbalance, training with weights can help your body overcome it. Frank took up archery for a while and found that one side of his body developed more than the other from continually pulling the bow on that side. Switching sides and using some additional weight-training movements helped balance this out.

There are some pieces of equipment that can be very useful in preventing injuries. One of the best and, we feel, essential pieces of equipment you can own when training with weights is a good lifting belt. When you buy one it should fit you exactly right, with very little overlap. The buckle should close in the front center. The belt should not be thick and wide in the front. You don't want it or the buckle digging into your waist when you bend forward. It should be comfortably wide in the rear for supporting your lower back, and the leather should be firm enough for support, but soft enough for comfort. The leather should be about 1/8 inch thick. This is the type of belt we find comfortable and wear when working out. Wear it when working all body parts except the waist, and wear it fairly tight. Remember that when you exercise you will expand a bit, and if your belt is too tight it will become even tighter after doing a set. You want to be comfortable yet feel supported at the same time.

If you do a lot of squatting movements, a pair of good elastic knee wraps will be helpful. (Wraps are sometimes used on the wrists when doing the Bench Press to give added support.) There is a brand of wraps called Elite or Super Wrap II which when wrapped around your knees moderately tightly can give a lot of spring to your squatting exercises, and help you to lift up. Never wrap your joints too tightly. When you do the exercise, your muscles get a "pump" and the size of the muscle increases. If you wrap too tightly you will be cutting off valuable blood. Begin wrapping below the knee at the top of your calf. Then cross over the knee and cross down behind the knee alternating several times. When you are near the end of the wrap, cover the space above the knee just at the base of your thigh. You will get a lot of movement in the knee area when you wrap this way and will not be putting any unnecessary pressure on the kneecap. If you wrap your elbows for any purpose, do it the same way as explained here for the knee. Remove knee wraps after each set of squats.

Often when your muscles are sore, you feel stiff and want to keep your muscles warm and loose during a workout. Taking a warm shower prior to your training period can help loosen you up, but the effects may not last long. We have found that using a liniment in these instances can be very helpful in relieving soreness and bringing warmth and circulation to the sore area. There are many preparations available for this purpose. Oil of wintergreen is natural and can be massaged sparingly into the muscle. It will heat up as you exercise and perspire. There are also many commercial preparations in liquid, cream and ointment form that create heat in the same manner. The liquid preparations can be merely applied to the area, but the creams and ointments should be massaged in well. Apply any type of preparation sparingly. The liniment will feel much hotter as time passes, so be careful not to put on too much. After you have applied this artificial heat, cover the area with a natural cloth such as a T-shirt or elastic-cotton wrap. For the elbows, we have found that a cotton or wool sock with the toes cut out slipped onto your arm to cover the elbow works very well. You'll get used to explaining to people why you are wearing your socks on your elbows!

Chiropractic

"The doctor of the future will give no medicine but will interest patients in the care of the human frame, in diet, and in the cause and prevention of disease."—Thomas Edison

Chiropractic is a system of adjusting segments of the spinal column and various other articulations of the body for restoration and maintenance of health. Our Chiropractor, Dr. E. L. Hexberg of Santa Monica, California—who quoted the above words of Thomas Edison to us—has been of tremendous help to us in preventing and treating injuries. The majority of injuries occur when you try to do too much, too soon or if you use too much weight and do the exercise incorrectly. One thing that can happen is mal-rotation of the vertebrae of the spinal column anywhere from the lower back up to the base of the skull. These mal-rotated vertebrae pinch off the foramen and put pressure on the nerve so that the muscle can't contract normally. This can cause strain or injury to the muscles involved, and these muscles won't pull or push in their usual channels. Mal-rotations to vertebrae can occur in exercises like Half Squat, Top Deadlift, Press Behind Neck, Incline Dumbbell Press or Barbell Row, when one side of the barbell (or one of the dumbbells) is raised before the other side. A twisted fifth lumbar vertebra is a common occurrence caused by coming up crooked in the Squat or Deadlift. Also, using a very wide grip and holding the bar with thumbs wrapped around it in exercises like Bench Press, Press Behind Back, Barbell Row, Wide-Grip Chins, or Wide-Grip Pulldowns can cause the forearms, wrists and elbows to pronate (turn excessively inward), throw the elbow joint out of alignment and cause pain in the forearm—elbow area. Supination, or twisting the wrist outward, can help correct this along with chiropractic elbow adjustments. The two uppermost vertebrae of the neck, the atlas and axis, can get mal-rotated or twisted in opposite directions from sleeping with the wrong pillow or other causes. When this happens, blackouts, dizziness, depression, headache, ocular disturbances and nausea may result. Muscle pain can also be caused by tannic acid from excessive drinking of coffee or tea. This can throw your body out of alignment.

Mal-rotations of vertebrae, excessive muscular soreness and other injuries seem to be more frequent during the first few weeks of any new exercise program. Whenever we have such problems we see our chiropractor immediately for an adjustment and sinusoidal current and/or ultra-sound therapy. Sinusoidal current is supplied by an electrical unit which contracts muscles without the individual exerting energy. During normal intense exercise, acids (products chiefly acid in nature, such as CO_2, lactic acid, pyruvic acids and acid phosphates known as fatigue substances) are stored in the muscles causing soreness. Sinusoidal current helps relieve this soreness (provided you don't keep the current on too long or too strong) because no energy is expended on your part. Soreness is relieved, and relaxation is induced because blood circulation is stepped up and some of the waste products are removed. For more severe muscle pulls or spasms, your chiropractor may use ultra sound which literally shakes the muscle cells by emitting up to one million vibrations per second. This causes the cells to excrete waste products and take on new nourishment. Ultra sound can cause a burn if used too long and should never be applied directly over eyes, spinal cord, nervous tissue, head or gonads.

The best way to choose a chiropractor is by referral. Ask experienced people who have a knowledge of exercise and nutrition. Also check with people who have had injuries and were helped by a chiropractor.

There are other things you can do to help prevent problems:

1. Don't cross your legs at the knee while sitting. This impairs circulation and distorts the pelvis.
2. Don't sit in big, soft chairs or divans. This can distort the pelvis and mal-rotate lumbar vertebrae.
3. Don't carry bulky objects in hip pockets.
4. Don't sleep near open windows. This can give you a stiff neck.

A chiropractor can help you, but since it is your body, it is your responsibility to keep your vertebrae and other body articulations in alignment by exercising regularly to keep the muscles well toned.

Many of the methods we mentioned that can be used for pleasurable sensations and enjoyment can also be used to heal an injured and sore body. Whirlpool and hydro-massage baths are really soothing and feel like a gentle massage. They can help increase your circulation and relax your muscles. Be sure that your water isn't too hot. A whirlpool bath for about 20 to 30 minutes at around 102 degrees Fahrenheit can really work wonders. If you don't have access to a whirlpool bath, try using a water shower-massage unit. They can be purchased just about anywhere now and are well worth the money, because they relax sore, tired muscles and increase the blood circulation. Use the shower massage everywhere on your body. Try using the pulsating jets on the soles of your feet and your toes. This kind of massage is very relaxing and works on the nerve endings which connect to all the parts of your anatomy from the feet. Spend about 10 minutes on each foot.

Hydroculators are another method of applying soothing heat to tense, sore muscles. They can be purchased at most drug stores. You place the hydroculator, which is a thick pad that retains heat for long periods of time, in a pan of boiling water following the directions on the box or insert. Next you fold a very thick towel several times (to prevent burning your skin) and lay this on the sore area. Now apply the hydroculator and cover with a natural cloth blanket or another thick towel. This will help retain the heat. If you are lying on top of it, place the hydroculator down first, then the folded towel. Now lie on top of it and place a blanket over yourself. Remain there about 20 minutes, or until the heat is nearly gone. The muscles will be very relaxed and loose when you get up. Keep the area warm and out of drafts, and cover with a natural cotton or wool cloth. Moist heat such as this penetrates much more deeply than dry heat. You will really feel the relief from this treatment.

Infra-red heat lamps can also be used to soothe sore, tight muscles. If you want the heat lamp to serve as a moist heat applicator, apply wet towels to the sore area and then turn the heat lamp on it. Don't place yourself too close to the lamp. About 12 to 18 inches is usually a good distance; but if the lamp is large, follow the directions that come with it. The results are not quite as good as with the hydroculator, but the heat lamp will relax you. Remain under the lamp for about 20 minutes. Heat lamps are not tanning lamps, so don't get them confused. You wouldn't want to stay under a tanning lamp for the same period of time. Check with a reliable, knowledgeable source when purchasing a bulb.

Another method to relieve your body's aches and pains is acupuncture. We explained a bit about acupressure points. Acupuncture works on the same points but with the use of fine needles. This technique should only be practiced by an experienced, licensed professional. It will relieve pain by hitting the nerves that control the pain centers. By learning the pressure points you can work on the same points without needles by using your hands. Massaging the points that are related to the sore area can help stimulate circulation and bring some relief. Get a good book on the subject or visit a professional for further guidance.

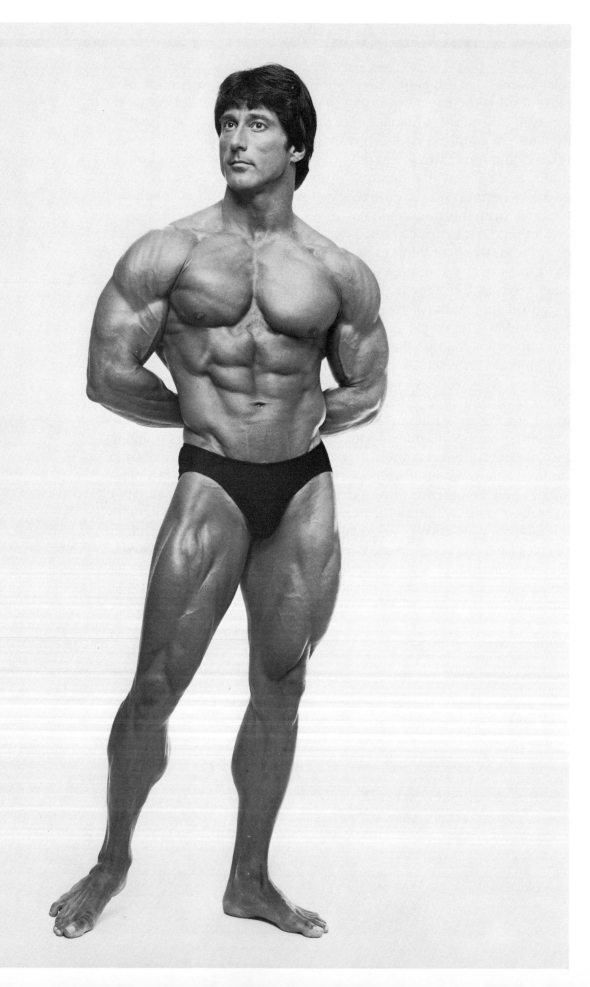

MEETING YOUR NUTRITIONAL NEEDS

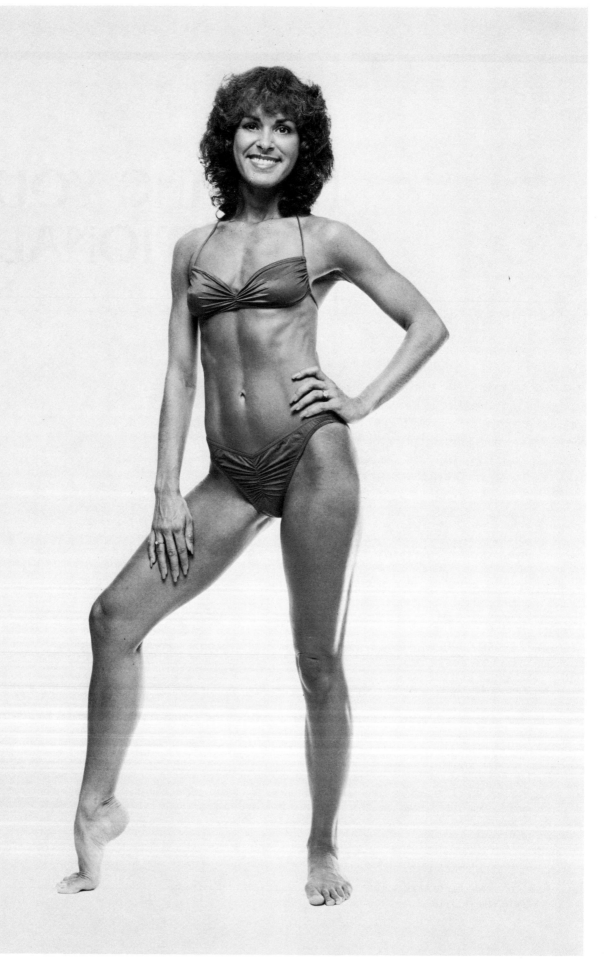

Diet and Menu Suggestions for Everyone's Needs

Your moods, how you feel physically and mentally, and certainly how you look are all partially determined by your diet and eating habits. You may be eating the right foods, but still are not able to lose weight. The right combinations, the correct amounts, and the time when the foods are eaten all play important parts in your overall health. In this section we have laid out menus for various diet goals. Whether you wish to build, trim or maintain your present body condition, there is a menu for you. Many people are light eaters, so we have included menus for them as well.

Our Typical Maintenance Diet

Here is an example of our maintenance diet for a typical day.

BREAKFAST
2 eggs (any style)
A few ounces of meat or cheese
½ to 1 piece of whole-grain bread or 2 salt-free Rye Krisp crackers
Butter
½ apple, ½ grapefruit, ½ cantaloupe or 1 cup strawberries (all in season)
Herb tea or 1 cup acid-free coffee

SNACK
6 ounces of fresh vegetable juice (carrot, tomato or a vegetable mix)

OR

1 ounce of cottage cheese mixed with fresh herbs

We don't have a snack if we're not hungry or if we ate too much the day before at our evening meal. If we feel that we can make it to lunch without feeling ravenous, then we skip the snack.

LUNCH

The snack above, with an ounce or two more of cottage cheese along with the juice, also provides a good lunch.

OR

1 piece of chicken
1 ounce of cheese or a 6- to 8-ounce glass of milk
Small salad or a piece of fruit
Sparkling mineral water with a twist of lemon or lime

Keep lunch small and allow for time to rest after you eat.

DINNER

4 to 6 ounces of broiled fish
medium to large mixed-greens salad with oil and vinegar

OR

Medium to medium-large amount of steamed low-carbohydrate vegetables
1 tablespoon mixture of sesame seeds and flaxseed
¾ cup grated salt-free cheese

⅛ small cantaloupe or 1 cup fresh strawberries
Sparkling mineral water and/or chamomile tea

We generally keep dinner light. We want to stay a little hungry for breakfast in the morning. If we overdo dinner, we end up having too much food to burn up and may not feel like eating in the morning when we really need the energy.

Vegetarians may wish to substitute tofu or other vegetable proteins for the animal proteins.

Choosing a Diet to Help You Reach Your Goal

Following are menus we would like you to use as examples of how to plan your eating. The meals will be basically the same whether you want to build, trim or maintain your body, but notice the subtle differences for accommodating both the building and the trimming physiques using basically the same foods.

The foods listed in the center and their amounts will give you an idea of a maintenance fitness program's ideals. Notice that it is much like the trimming menu. Use the build category to gain size, the trim to reduce and the average category to maintain.

BREAKFAST

Build
3-egg omelet—filling: chicken, spinach and ricotta cheese
1 small apple—garnish with cinnamon
1 slice whole-grain bread
Herb tea

Average
2 eggs (any style)
½ chicken breast
¼ cup spinach
⅛ slice cantaloupe
1 tablespoon yogurt
Herb tea

Trim
2 eggs (any style)
2 slices chicken breast
½ slice whole-grain toast
1 teaspoon butter (unsalted)
Herb tea

LUNCH

2–3 cups homemade chicken soup (lots of meat)
Steamed low-carbohydrate vegetables
Garnish soup with 1 tablespoon sour cream
1 cup milk, yogurt or cottage cheese
¼ honeydew melon
Mineral water

1 cup chicken soup (mostly broth and onion)
3–4 ounces chicken meat
1 cup steamed low-carbohydrate vegetables
1 Rye Krisp with 1 ounce cheese melted on top
Mineral water or 1 cup low-fat milk
½ apple

Chicken soup (broth)
1½ cups low-carbohydrate steamed vegetables
1 Rye Krisp with 1 ounce melted cheese
Sparkling mineral water
1/16 cantaloupe or honeydew melon

DINNER

10 ounces broiled seafood
Slaw made from scallion, zucchini, mushroom, tomato, oil, vinegar, pepper and dry mustard
½ papaya
½ cup protein drink made very thick and poured over papaya
Chamomile tea

3–4 ounces broiled seafood
1–1½ cups slaw (see Build column)
½ papaya
½ cup plain yogurt
Chamomile tea

1 large vegetable salad
½ cup seafood added to salad
¼ papaya with 1 teaspoon sour cream
Chamomile tea

Diet Suggestions for Days When You Are Less Active and for Those Who Prefer to Eat Light Meals

Each week in your program you have a day of rest from training. Since you will be doing less physically, you should also eat less.

This first menu is divided into Build and Trim categories. A diet between these two would be for maintenance. You will notice that there are more carbohydrates, so keep your portions small. Following these suggestions will give you the amount of energy that you will need for your workout the following day. Small amounts of complex carbohydrates stay with you longer and provide a lot of energy. Also, eat more slowly.

Raw foods are excellent for taking to work. Put them in air-tight containers or take them uncut and eat them whole or freshly sliced at your office. Here are some of our suggestions for light eating. Try one meal or all three.

BREAKFAST
Have all ingredients at room temperature and in their freshest, natural, raw state. Use this menu whether you want to build, trim or maintain.
1 slice unleavened sprouted-wheat bread
Spread bread with 2 ounces Camembert cheese.
Top the cheese with 1 tablespoon pureed banana and cinnamon.
Garnish with 1 tablespoon raw sunflower seeds.
Pink Mint herb tea (a mix of hibiscus and peppermint)

Those who want to build may also have an 8-ounce serving of plain yogurt mixed with freshly made apple sauce (no additives).

LUNCH
1 cup of protein ice cream for those who want to gain and ¾ cup for those who want to lose. (See recipe section for ice cream.)
One tablespoon chopped raw pecans or almonds, only for those who want to build. 1 cup fresh, in season, low-carbohydrate fruit or a mixture of fruits to serve over the ice cream.

The ice cream can be taken to work in a thermos and eaten like a thick pudding.

Those who want to gain weight may have a second portion after waiting at least 10 minutes. Eat this meal very slowly; it requires ample time to digest. You may like to freeze this ice cream in cups with sticks inserted so that it can be eaten like an ice-cream bar. We like it best in a bowl with toppings mixed in. For those who love yogurt, it can be made with yogurt instead of cream. Or better yet, substitute yogurt for the milk in the recipe and keep the cream in. The texture is creamier with cream and icier without it.

DINNER
Make a raw salad like the Raw Health Salad with Lemon Dressing described in the recipe section.

Sometimes you will want a lighter menu but one lower in carbohydrates than the previous one. The following suggestions for light meals are very appropriate for you to follow when you are in the Intermediate and Advanced portions of the weight-training program.

Refrain from adding salt to your foods. This masks the taste and somewhat numbs your taste buds. After a while all you seem to taste is salt. You may have to reeducate your taste buds before you can fully enjoy the variety of tastes present in fresh, natural foods that are eaten without salt. It is essential for your health that you drop salt from your food list.

In the Intermediate and Advanced programs your meals should contain fewer and fewer simple-sugar and high-carbohydrate foods. Limit the amounts as well as the frequency with which you eat them. If you are eating ice cream (of course the protein ice cream we suggested) a great deal, and you are in the Advanced Program, then you should begin limiting the amount, and have it only in the morning, every other day or every third day. This should help you progress more quickly. Keep juggling and working with the foods that you eat, the amounts and even the time of day when you are eating until you find what works best for you. You will learn more about the responses your body gives to different situations and food combinations. This is one way your food record can help you tremendously.

Here are some lighter meals for those interested in building or trimming and who want to lower the amount of carbohydrates in their diet.

BREAKFAST

Build
3 poached or soft-boiled eggs served atop a slice of whole-grain toast.
2 teaspoons butter
½ cup homemade apple sauce
2 ounces cheese
Herb tea

Trim
2 poached or soft-boiled eggs on whole-wheat toast
1 teaspoon butter
½ cup homemade apple sauce
1 ounce cheese
Herb tea

LUNCH

4 ounces fresh broiled fish
Serve a mix of mayonnaise, cottage cheese, grated Swiss cheese, and chopped chives with the fish.
½ medium-sized fresh peach
Sparkling mineral water

3 ounces fresh broiled fish
Serve lemon and butter with fish.
Mixed-greens salad with lemon and yogurt as a dressing
Sparkling mineral water

DINNER

4 ounces any hard cheese
Large salad of mixed greens and low-carbohydrate vegetables, with ½ cup of leftover meat or fish, and 2 hard-boiled eggs.
Use the dressing on the trim menu.
Iced mint tea

Medium-size salad of mixed greens and low-carbohydrate vegetables
Dressing: Mix paprika, dry mustard, pepper, oil, vinegar, celery or caraway seed, and flaxseed.
Iced mint tea

Optional for both: 1 to 2 whole-wheat bread sticks

Whether you want to build or trim or just maintain your physique, always make breakfast your heartiest meal, with lunch a little smaller and dinner the smallest meal of all—and always check the nutritive values of the foods you eat.

Competition Diet

For those who may be preparing for physique competition, we have included the following low-carbohydrate/high-protein menu.

A diet such as this should be followed only with the approval of your doctor, and for not more than three or four weeks prior to a serious competition where minimum body fat is essential. Since it is extremely low in carbohydrates (under 20 grams) it could cause lethargy and vertigo, especially in those with hypoglycemia. This type of diet is used to help a bodybuilder show more muscularity by getting rid of all excess fat. Most of the carbohydrates taken in are complex carbohydrates (starches) and are best utilized when eaten early in the day and prior to workouts. If lethargy and vertigo occur, complex carbohydrates should be increased to 40 grams per day for a short period of time. Eating no later than 7 P.M. and some kind of physical activity in the evening also help to accelerate the fat-burning process.

The following example of how we have dieted is only a suggestion of menus to follow. Everyone's needs are different and all diets should be adapted to fit your needs and schedules.

Quantities are only important where a specific amount is indicated. But remember that it is never wise to stuff yourself and stretch your stomach. If you are still hungry after a meal, wait an hour or so and have a small protein snack. The number in parentheses indicates the approximate amount of carbohydrate grams.

BREAKFAST
Eggs any style
½ avocado (7 grams) or ½ potato (7 to 10 grams)
Optional: butter
Beef
Herb Tea

LUNCH
Fresh fish, no breading or batters
Mixed green salad (8 to 10 grams)
Oil and vinegar for salad
Herb tea or sparkling mineral water

DINNER
Fresh fowl, no breading or batter
Herb tea or sparkling mineral water

PRE-WORKOUT SNACK

One hour before workout

2 to 3 soft-boiled eggs *or* 3 to 4 ounces low sodium cheese

Read all labels to be sure you aren't getting any added carbohydrates through sugars (sucrose, dextrose, lactose, fructose, etc.) or starches. Try to avoid all salt. You'll find some mineral waters contain more sodium than others. Club soda is generally very high in sodium.

Most people will begin responding to a diet like this in about a week's time. The result will be a thinning out of the fat layer under the skin and a more visible muscular appearance.

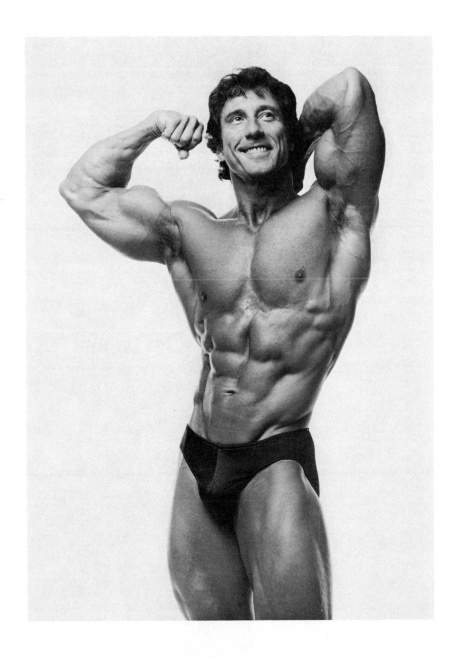

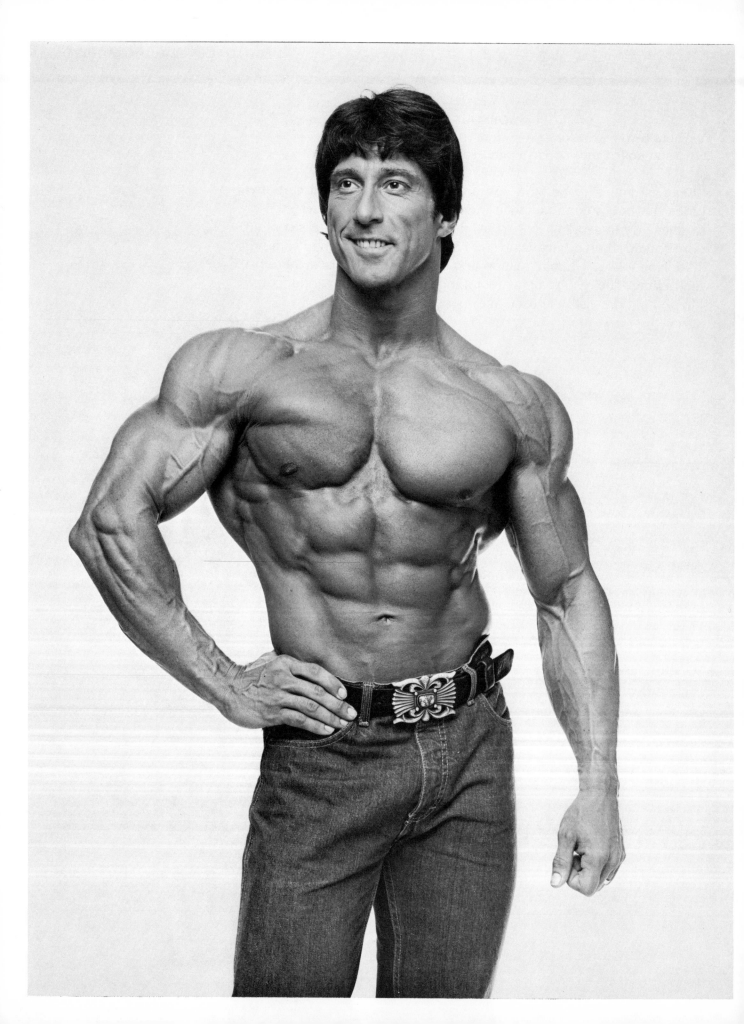

COOKING
HEALTHY

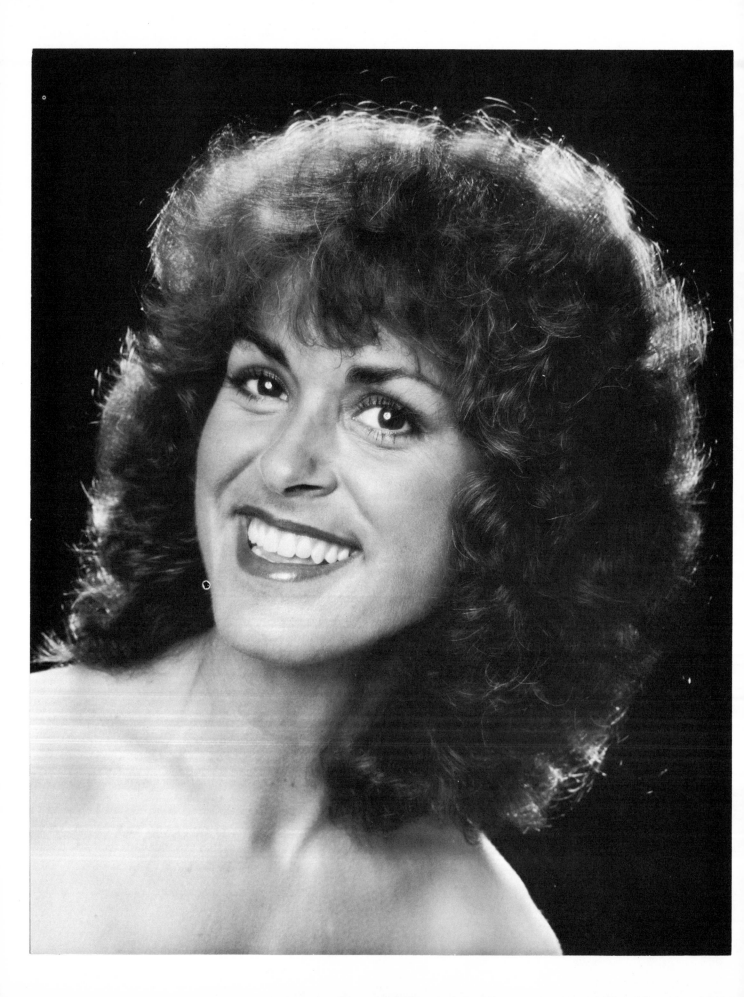

Technique

We'll cover the methods we have used to prepare our healthy meals and give you some suggestions for meals and some of our favorite recipes.

The easiest and healthiest method of food preparation is no preparation—serving fresh, raw foods. The less you do to your food, the better it is. Not all foods can be eaten raw, therefore we offer the following alternatives: steaming, baking, broiling and, last, frying.

Steamed foods are extremely flavorful and juicy. All foods can be steamed: fruits, vegetables, meat, fish and poultry. Steaming cooks food at a lower temperature with moist heat. The juices don't escape and the flavor isn't boiled out with water. Steaming vegetables breaks down the cellulose and makes the food easier to digest. Light steaming allows some of the cellulose to be broken down and some to remain as bulk in the diet (fiber). More of the vitamins and minerals, in fact, are retained this way than with any other cooking method. Put some herbs, lemon slices or a clove of fresh garlic in your steaming pot to add flavor to vegetables or meats.

There are many steaming containers available on the market today. There is a steamer basket which easily fits inside almost any size pot; or you can use the stackable steamer trays, made of bamboo or stainless steel. If you have a wok you can get a steaming rack, which you place your plate on inside the wok. A large sieve or strainer can serve to hold your food and be propped up in a pot. Just make certain in any method you use that the water doesn't touch the food. We like the ceramic steamer which is placed on a pot of boiling water; the steam rises in a short chimney in the center of the steamer and hits the lid instead of directly contacting the food. We feel more nutrients are retained with this type of pot. It cost a little more than a steaming basket or a strainer, but good utensils are what cooking good food is all about. A device like this pays for itself many times over with the amount of use we get out of it, as well as the amount of nutrition we save from being poured down the drain.

Baking your foods is another healthy way to prepare them. It is a dry-heat method of cooking and a moist method of cooking combined. The oven heat is dry and the natural juices create a vapor which circulates and surrounds the food being baked. Fruits, vegetables, grains and meats can be baked. We prefer to use terra-cotta stone baking utensils along with the glass and metal pans.

You can cook your food without adding fat, and it browns nicely and stays moist and succulent. Bread stays moist and forms a wonderful brown crust in terra-cotta.

Broiling and frying are two methods of cooking that we are sure you are familiar with. Broiling is done under a heat source, and sometimes the food is brushed with oil. Frying is done in oil or some sort of fat and can add many unnecessary calories to your diet. Frying usually requires some type of batter to form the flaky, brown crust on fried chicken, fish or tempura vegetables. This batter is often made from flour, water and eggs and adds empty calories and carbohydrates. If you fry foods, do so in a skillet with a nonstick surface without adding fats or batters. Broiling is a much better method of preparing your food. It can be done on a grill or in the oven. This is a dry heat that can be adjusted by moving the rack either closer, if you want to cook the outside faster than the inside (as in rare and medium-rare), or farther away from the heat source for more thorough interior cooking. Preheat your broiling unit, but always place food on a cold rack (to prevent sticking) and make sure there is proper ventilation. We prefer the Farberware broiler; the heat source is adjustable and the fat drips down to a tray so your food doesn't sit in fat while cooking, nor does it smoke and smell. Never allow food to sit in the fat while cooking.

Breakfast Breaks

Breakfast is exactly that . . . the time when you break the fast you have been on since yesterday evening's meal. If you are not used to eating a good breakfast and find it either too much trouble to fix or not too appetizing to eat, you might try a lighter high-protein meal. If you want to gain weight (not fat), have a good 10-ounce serving of the following recipe, and if you are working toward being slimmer have an 8-ounce glass. It is easily prepared in a blender, with a rotary mixer, or shaken in a closed container, in a minimum of time. It can even be made ahead, but tastes best when fresh. Follow the directions under the appropriate category, according to your needs.

Build	Trim
1 cup whole milk, half-and-half or plain kefir or yogurt	1 cup nonfat or skim milk

Have your blender going at medium speed and add:

Build	Trim
¼ cup vanilla milk egg protein powder	Same as Build
2 drops pure vanilla	Same as Build
2 raw eggs	Same as Build
½ cup fresh strawberries or 1 medium plum, with ½ banana	Same choice as Build but NO banana
Top with toasted wheat germ	Sprinkle with cinnamon

Pour into well-chilled attractive soda style glasses. Sip the drink slowly. It contains a great deal of nutrition and is digested more easily this way. Have the ingredients on hand in case you don't have a lot of time to prepare your meal. It doesn't only have to be for breakfast.

This is a recipe for those of you who, like us, take the time to prepare a substantial breakfast and really do enjoy it. We like variety and believe you should eat the foods you enjoy at times other than when they are traditionally served. For example, bacon, eggs and toast make a very good dinner as well as a favorite breakfast. Mixed Grill is a recipe which pleases every taste. It can consist of just about any combination of meats and vegetables. They are all prepared on a grill or broiled in your oven. If fried eggs accompany the grill, prepare them separately without added fat. The portions should be small, and the selection varied. Mixed Grill is best prepared for more than one person, but both those interested in building and trimming can have this breakfast. Those on a trimming diet should eat slowly, choose a wide variety (you don't have to eat everything) and keep the portions small.

Mixed Grill Choices
Broiled tomato halves with cheese topping
Broiled or grilled mushrooms brushed with butter
Bacon
Sausage
Broiled liver
Broiled pork chops
Broiled chicken wings
Broiled lamb chops
Eggs
Onions broiled and stuffed with cheese
Yams sliced diagonally, brushed with butter and grilled (Build only)
Serve the Mixed Grill with:
Thinly sliced whole-grain, unleavened pumpernickel bread with butter (one piece only)

Fresh grapefruit sections (½ grapefruit for Build and ¼ grapefruit for Trim)
Milk (Build only), herb tea for beverage

If there are a lot of people eating with you, prepare more variety. If only you and one other person are eating, prepare less, maybe six items out of the listed foods. Serve everything from the same platter. Have the foods in separate sections and attractively displayed. Decorate the plate with some edible greens or herbs.

Salads

When you select ingredients for a salad keep in mind what your goal is and which foods will help you reach it. If you wish to gain weight you might choose from the following: avocados, corn (very fresh), various sprouted grains (can be pressed together and eaten as a bread or added to salad and eaten like a vegetable), raw nuts (in moderation), fresh peas, bananas, peaches, cherries, carrots, pears and all the foods which follow for those who want to trim. Of course, all foods should be fresh, not canned or frozen. For trimming choose from: leafy vegetables (spinach, lettuce, dandelion greens), strawberries, grapefruit, melon, tomatoes, green onions, red onions, red and green peppers, mushrooms, plums, flaxseed, yellow squash, zucchini and summer squash.

Choose foods that have a great deal of variety in taste, texture and appearance. Appeal to sour or tart taste buds as well as sweet. Dilute the stronger tasting foods (like turnip and beet) by shredding, slicing or grating them, and combining them with weaker, more subtle flavors (like lettuce and sprouts). Combine crisp, crunchy foods with more tender ones. Make your salad a work of art, inviting you to enjoy it. Take into consideration the colors of the food—use a variety of reds, yellows and greens to give your meal a vibrant, alive look. It's much easier to eat food that is attractive and appealing.

Wash, drain and dry the salad ingredients quickly. They can be stored (uncut) in a cloth sack (like a cotton pillow case) in the refrigerator to keep them chilled, crisp and dry. Keep the salad cold until time to serve it, and don't add the dressing until you are ready to eat. If you serve a wide variety of the freshest ingredients possible in a salad you may find there is no need for a dressing at all. Salads can be served not only as meal accompaniment but as a main course, a snack, vegetable or dessert. For a salad higher in protein we suggest adding a small amount of cottage cheese, grated hard-cooked egg, meat, chicken or fish.

The following recipe is one of our main course salad variations that we are sure you'll like.

RAW HEALTH SALAD
Arrange the following foods in a bowl or platter in a pleasing manner:

½ cup cauliflower floweret, separated in ½–1-inch sections

½ cup broccoli floweret, separated into ½–1-inch sections

½ red onion sliced very thin and separated into rings

¼ bunch of watercress

¼ cup of grated raw beet

1 cup mung bean sprouts

½ cup garbanzo bean sprouts (chick peas)

½ cup carrots cut thinly on the diagonal

½ salad bowl, which serves two people, of spinach leaves.

½ cubed avocado

½ teaspoon each: raw sunflower seeds, sesame seeds, flaxseed.

   Serve with your choice of the following dressings: (Toss lightly; don't drown the salad in dressing.)

LEMON DRESSING
1 tablespoon fresh lemon juice

small amount of onion puree or juice

½ tablespoon peanut oil

a small amount of water

   Mix all of the above well in a shaker or blend with a wire whisk or in the blender.

YOGURT DRESSING
Blend together your choice from the following:

Yogurt and celery seed

Yogurt and paprika (or other natural spice)

Yogurt and garlic (fresh garlic pressed to get the juice)

Yogurt and chopped green pepper

   Use only additive-free, plain (not flavored) yogurt.

COTTAGE CHEESE DRESSING
8 ounces cottage cheese (low-fat or whole)

½ teaspoon fresh lemon juice

2 teaspoons grated lemon rind (none that has been sprayed or colored)

½ teaspoon freshly ground ginger

   Blend well and serve chilled.

BLUE CHEESE DRESSING
¼ cup crumbled blue cheese

2 tablespoons fresh lemon juice

1 cup sour cream

½ teaspoon dry mustard

½ teaspoon paprika

   Blend together and adjust to fit your tastes. Serve chilled. (Blue cheese should remain a little chunky; do not blend it too smoothly.)

OIL AND VINEGAR
¾ cup oil (peanut, garlic-flavored, or olive oil)
½ cup white vinegar (flavored with herbs)
　　Add to the salad in portions that please you or mix together well and serve.

Vegetables

There are a variety of ways to prepare vegetables. Marinate raw vegetables in your favorite marinade and serve them chilled or at room temperature. Steam and toss them in a mixture of hot butter and your favorite herbs and spices, or an herb and plain yogurt or sour cream mixture. Steamed vegetables are good served either hot or cold.

　　If you are having a baked protein dish, consider baking your vegetables along with it. This will give them a roasted taste, which is a bit different than steamed. Preparing them in individual ways adds variety to your meals even if you're eating the same foods. When you combine foods that you enjoy, and bake them in one dish, their flavors mingle and create a new taste. We've seen people who have sworn that they hate a certain vegetable, but when it is baked in combination with a food they like, they really rave about how delicious it is! When you tell them that it's "that vegetable you hate," they won't believe it.

　　Here is a recipe for a baked dish which is full of flavor and nutrition and very low in calories and carbohydrates.

TOMATOES AND ONIONS CASSEROLE
　　Slice all the following vegetables and toss them in 1 tablespoon of melted butter until well coated.
1 onion
2 firm red tomatoes (peeled)
¼ cup chopped fresh parsley
　　Arrange these ingredients in a well-oiled and buttered casserole dish and cover with grated cheese (about 2–3 tablespoons). Bake in a 350-degree, preheated oven for 30 minutes. Serve while it is hot.

　　Other good vegetable and cheese combinations are zucchini, tomatoes and ricotta cheese; eggplant, onions, with mozzarella cheese; or you can combine your favorite vegetable or vegetables with cheese of your choice and create your own masterpiece.

Beef

We like our beef prepared very simply, either broiled or slow baked, preferably without sauces and whole, not ground.

Poultry

Poultry is such a versatile food and it tastes deliciously different each way you prepare it. Each of the following recipes has a new and exciting flavor.

1. Rotisserie—spit broiled. Stuff with oranges and onions. Rub the inside and outside with one of the orange quarters before stuffing. After cooked, don't eat the stuffing. Garnish with freshly grated orange rind. Cook according to spit directions that come with your rotisserie.
2. Baked—using a clay baking container. Peel and slice a lemon thinly. Place these slices under the skin of the poultry. Using a sharp, pointed object, poke holes in the skin and insert whole cloves in a pattern, spacing them about ½ inch apart. Don't eat the cloves but do leave them on when serving, for beauty. Baking time will vary according to size.
3. Foil baked—in a slow oven (250–300 degrees). Use herb combinations of your choice and rub into the outside and into the cavity of the poultry. Place it on a raised rack in a baking dish so that it doesn't sit in fat. Cover with foil and cook slowly until done. It should take longer at lower temperatures. Don't prick the skin. Instead, move the leg back and forth. If it feels as though the bone can be removed easily or fall off, it is done.
4. Steamed. This method will keep the fowl juicy. To prepare steamed poultry, place it on a steaming rack, in a pot where the steam can circulate easily around it. Add herbs and any of the following liquids to the water to flavor the fowl. Amounts depend on the size of your pot.

   Beer, onion, bay leaf and whole peppercorns
   Distilled water, apple juice, cinnamon stick, whole cloves
   Distilled water, garlic bulbs (cut), lemon slices (skinless)
   Distilled water, orange juice, cinnamon, mint leaves
   White wine, onions, peppercorns.

Or you may want to toss the poultry pieces in your favorite herbs and/or add vegetables or sprouts during the last 5 minutes of steaming and have your entire dinner from one pot.

While steaming, keep the lid on tightly, unless adding ingredients, checking water or rearranging your food to cook evenly. Cook it the same length of time as you would roast it in an oven. Check your cookbook for the number of minutes required.

Fish

Fish is as versatile as chicken, when it comes to adding various flavors. Some fish are stronger than others in taste, some are firmer and have less fat content than others. Check with a reputable fresh fish market in your area. If it is possible, stick with fish that are caught locally. They will be lower in cost and fresher. Fresh fish tastes so much better than frozen. One fish that you don't want to eat is the fish that has been prepared by a fast-food establishment. It is frozen, breaded (usually more bread than fish) and salted excessively. Eat fish prepared without all the unnecessary breading and batters.

Did you try the steamed chicken (or other fowl)? Steamed fish is just as tasty. We recommend using a firm, meaty fish, such as red snapper, shark, swordfish or halibut. Fish like cod and sole tend to be too soft and fall apart when cooking. Steam it whole or in fillets, or chunks. The steaming time will be the same as for baked fish. Fish flakes easily when it is done, and use a fork to gently make the doneness test. Steam the fish in the same way that you steamed the fowl. Fish adapts to many different flavors. Make a marinade from oil, vinegar, dry mustard and herbs and marinate your fish before cooking. When removing the fish from your steamer, do so carefully. Fish is very delicate and falls apart more readily after it is cooked. You may wish to lay down a bed of fresh spinach (or other greens) under the fish before steaming so that it can be easily lifted out of the pan by the greens. Smaller pieces can be removed with a large, slotted spoon.

Try baking fish in a covered container, after being marinated or brushed with melted butter and fresh herbs. You can also add cheese and vegetables for variation.

Have you ever had poached fish? You can get a fish poacher, which has a perforated tray allowing the fish to be lowered into and lifted out of the liquid it is being poached in. When poaching fish, you want it to be constantly bathed in liquid, so don't crowd the fish in the pan. It will only take about 8 to 10 minutes to cook, depending on the size of the portions. Poach in white wine, dairy products, lemon water with white peppercorns and a bay leaf or a fish stock with finely chopped vegetables.

Fish is also very good fixed on skewers like kebobs, or cut into cubes and sauteed or stir-fried in a wok.

If you would like to prepare light fish dishes for your rest day, try cold salmon or other fish with herb mayonnaise, yogurt or sour cream or try the recipe that follows for Fish Mousse.

FISH MOUSSE
1 pound of sole or flounder fillets
1 cup cream
dash of cayenne pepper
¼ teaspoon chopped fresh dill weed
2 eggs, separated
4 tablespoons butter
¼ to ½ cup wheat germ flakes

Blend, in a bowl, the fillets and ½ cup cream to a paste consistency. Add wheat germ and seasonings. Beat the egg whites until stiff and fold very gently into the fish mixture. Pour into a buttered loaf pan or a fish mold and cover with foil. Place in another pan of hot water and bake in a preheated 325-degree oven for 1 hour or until nicely firm. Remove from the oven and let sit for 10 to 12 minutes. Unmold on a serving plate. To make a sauce, use the other ½ cup of cream and the egg yolks and beat together until smooth and lemony colored. Stir in butter and heat it over low heat. Pour over the mousse. You may want to use less butter.

Cheese and Eggs

These recipes use low-calorie, low-carbohydrate, high-nutrition foods for delicious, satisfying results. Use only good ricotta (from a cheese shop or Italian market), real cottage cheese and real cheeses. None should contain any additives, preservatives or fillers.

RICOTTA PIE

Beat together 2 eggs, 1 tablespoon finely chopped onion, 3 ounces grated mozzarella cheese, 1 teaspoon fresh parsley that has been chopped, ¼ teaspoon oregano or an Italian herb mixture, 1 pound of ricotta cheese (fresh) and a little freshly ground pepper. Pour this mixture into a baking dish that has been well oiled with olive oil. Top with 3 more ounces of grated mozzarella cheese and add ¼ cup of freshly grated Parmesan cheese. Bake in a preheated oven at 325 degrees for 1 hour. Serve hot.

CHEESEY CUSTARD (with NO sugar!)

Scald 1 cup milk. Gradually stir in 4 eggs that have been slightly beaten. Now add, while still stirring, 1¼ cups grated cheddar cheese (sharp) and a dash of cayenne pepper. When thoroughly mixed, pour into custard cups or a small pan and place in a baking pan that contains 1 inch of water. Bake in a preheated 350-degree oven for 30 minutes. It will be done when you can insert a knife and it comes out clean.

JELLY-EGG ROLL

Have prepared in advance some fruit jam (see dessert section). Prepare enough to spread generously on the size of egg roll that you plan to make. The following recipe will serve one. Have ready a well-oiled, rectangular pan with sides. Using a blender, blend thoroughly 2 eggs, 2 teaspoons soy flour, ¼ cup nonfat dry milk and a dash of cinnamon. Pour this mixture into the pan. It should be thin, about ⅛ to ¼ inch deep. Bake for a few minutes in a 350-degree oven. When the egg mixture is almost done, not quite set on top, slide it onto a sheet of wax paper and spread it with jam, about ⅛ inch thick. Lifting the paper from one end, begin forming the egg mixture into a roll. It's easier to roll if you wait for it to cool just slightly. After rolling, it will continue to cook and firm, so don't allow it to cool so much that it won't properly firm. Place the roll, seam down, on a clean plate and garnish with mint leaves and fresh fruit. If you prepare a large roll to serve several people, cut it into 1-inch slices and serve on individual, garnished plates.

FRIED CHEESE

Cut a wheel of Camembert or Brie, which is not fully ripened, into triangular pieces. Dredge them in a little flour and dip into a mixture of egg and milk (1 egg, 1 tablespoon milk). Next, dip the cheese into dry bread crumbs.

Repeat the dip into the egg and milk, and again the bread crumbs. (You could substitute dry onion flakes for the bread crumbs.) Melt some butter in a skillet and sauté the cheese until golden brown and crisp on both sides. Serve immediately. When you cut into the cheese it will lusciously ooze out of its crust.

This same method can be used to prepare mozzarella, Edam, Gouda or any semi-soft cheese. We really like mozzarella because it's so low in calories and fats. We often fry mozzarella without a coating, but you have to be very careful not to overcook it, and very careful when you turn it over. Add some sesame or flaxseed to the cheese fixed this way. It's really delicious.

Bread

We are sure that a lot of you bread lovers really dislike the thought of giving up bread, so we know you'll enjoy these recipes. They are a cinch to make, taste surprisingly good and are lower in both carbohydrates and calories than conventional bread. The recipe for gluten bread is one of our favorites. It's a yeast bread, and its taste can be altered by kneading in different spices and seeds.

BASIC GLUTEN BREAD

Have all your ingredients at room temperature (about 75 degrees), unless otherwise specified. You will need two 5- by 9-inch loaf pans. (Using terracotta pans gives this bread a real countrylike, stone-oven crust.) In a bowl, combine 3 cups of warm water (85 degrees) and one crumbled cake or packet of yeast. Allow this to stand until dissolved (about 10 minutes). Using a wire wisk (or fork), beat in 2 cups of unsifted gluten flour. Let this sit for about 30 minutes or until light and frothy. Use a wire whisk or a large spoon and beat in a mixture of 1 egg (beaten), 2 tablespoons melted butter, ½ teaspoon salt and 1 teaspoon raw sugar. (The salt and raw sugar activate the yeast to help raise the bread.) Use a large spoon to stir in about 3½ cups more flour and 4 tablespoons flaxseed. Don't use more flour than you need to obtain a good texture for kneading the bread. Save some flour for your kneading board. When the bread dough begins to leave the sides of the bowl, you can turn it onto a lightly floured board. Use a plastic pastry board with a slight texture, and you'll have no problems with sticking. Flour your hands lightly before you begin kneading. Knead for five minutes. This is the time to add other herbs, spices and flavors. Choose from the following: (Since this recipe makes two loaves, you might divide the dough and make two different flavors.)

Cinnamon powder—roll the dough into a rectangle and brush with melted butter. Sprinkle generously with cinnamon and roll up to fit your pan.

Dill seeds
Celery seed
Sunflower seeds

Chopped nuts
Caraway seeds—for a rye taste
Leftover steamed vegetables—chopped finely
Grated cheddar cheese—½ cup per loaf
Chopped onion

You may use a combination of any of the above but don't overload the bread. You want to keep it light.

After kneading, form the dough into two loaves and place into clay pans (bread won't stick to them) or lightly oiled regular pans. Let rise in a draft-free, warm place until double in bulk. Meanwhile, preheat oven to 350 degrees. When ready place in the oven and bake for 1 hour. About 15 minutes before they are done you may wish to brush the tops with egg white and sprinkle on sesame, poppy or caraway seeds. When done, remove the bread by tapping the bottom of the pan gently and place them on a rack to cool thoroughly before wrapping. To test for doneness, tap the bottom of the loaves; if the sound is hollow and the bread is nicely browned, they are done. If the sound isn't hollow, they need to be returned to the oven and baked a bit longer.

The following breads are less like bread and more like muffins in texture. No yeast or kneading is required. Serve with your favorite topping, such as melted cheese, alfalfa sprouts or avocado.

SOY BREAD

1 cup full fatted soy flour
½ cup milk
6 eggs, separated
¼ teaspoon salt
⅓ cup dry nonfat milk

Beat egg yolks with all other ingredients except egg whites. In a separate bowl, beat egg whites until they form stiff peaks. Fold egg whites into the other mixture and mix. Pour this into a loaf pan. Preheat oven and bake at 350 degrees for about 45 minutes or until set. Cool before cutting.

Beating the egg whites makes a lighter bread. If you don't have the time to do this, you can mix all ingredients at the same time. Add minced onion, caraway seeds or cinnamon and a drop or two of artificial sweetener (if you don't mind using it).

SOY-CREAM BISCUITS

1¼ cups soy flour (full fatted)
½ pint heavy cream (no sugars, preservatives or additives)
1 teaspoon baking powder

Blend well. Butter your hands so the batter doesn't stick to you, and form the dough into small balls about 1½ inches in diameter. Place in a flat pan about 1–1½ inches apart. Bake in a preheated oven at 425 degrees for about 10 minutes or until golden brown. This will make a few dozen biscuits, depending on their size.

Desserts

Our first recipe treat can be the filling for your Jelly-Egg Roll or a delicious spread for the bread and muffin recipes. It's a jam, but it doesn't contain sugar!

STRAWBERRY JAM
1 envelope strawberry dietetic gelatin (or if you prefer no artificial ingredients, use 1 envelope gelatin)
1 cup water
1 pint ripe, fresh strawberries (A bit more if you wish.)
   Cook all of these ingredients over medium heat until they come to a slow boil. Stir and mash down while cooking. Remove from the heat and let it sit. When cool, put into jars and refrigerate. You can even freeze this for times when strawberries are hard to come by.
   A variation on the above recipe can be made with ripe peaches, blackberries or blueberries. With blueberries use a teaspoon of lemon juice and with all of these fruits use plain gelatin. If you are accustomed to the overly sweet, almost pure sugar, jams you buy in the stores, you may have to get used to the fresh, natural fruit taste of these new jams. They are delicious and a welcome addition to every breakfast.

YOGURT FREEZE
Mix to taste the following:
1 cup plain yogurt
¼ teaspoon vanilla bean or pure extract
1 tablespoon orange or ½ tablespoon lemon juice
1 cup strwaberries
   Blend well and freeze. Before eating, let stand in the refrigerator until soft enough to eat.

PROTEIN ICE CREAM
1 cup cream (no additives)	1 cup whole milk
1 cup fresh ripe peaches (pureed)	1 teaspoon vanilla bean or extract
1 raw egg	1 cup protein powder (milk-egg-based Blair's Protein is excellent)

   Combine and freeze. Serve when left to soften in refrigerator.
   Those who want to lose weight or those who are maintaining should eat small amounts only (¼ cup).
   This ice-cream recipe was given to us by nutritionist Rheo H. Blair, Los Angeles, CA.

BERRIES AND CREAM
2 to 3 cups strawberries (ripe and in season)	¼ cup heavy cream
	2 egg whites
1 teaspoon almond extract	

   Beat the egg whites until stiff peaks form. Whip the cream until it holds peaks. Mix egg whites with almond extract. Fold this mixture into the cream. Layer berries and cream, alternating to fill fancy dessert glasses.

You may want to try baking some fruit. These are very good in cold weather and are a satisfying change of pace for breakfast or dessert. Rome Beauty apples, bananas (in moderation) and peaches all are excellent for baking. Add spices, cream or citrus juice to the fruit.

Snacks

Often you just don't feel like sitting down to a full meal and would rather snack. As long as you don't overeat, this is fine. The following recipes can be eaten as snack-meals throughout the day, or for light snacks on just about any day; or they can be taken to work or school as lunch. Snacking can add variety to your style of eating. The following recipes are meant to be served in small portions.

LIVER PÂTÉ
(Makes about 8 snack servings. Keep refrigerated.)
1 pound chicken livers (hormone and preservative free)
1 chopped white onion
1 tablespoon heavy cream
¼ teaspoon coarsely ground pepper
⅛ teaspoon ground thyme
⅛ teaspoon ground bay leaf
2 egg yolks
unsalted butter

Sauté onions in a little butter until brown and clear. Pour this into a blender with the juices from the pan. Now, cook the chicken livers with a little butter until brown on the outside and pink inside. Put them in the blender with the onions. Begin blending at a slow speed and gradually increase to high speed. Add the remainder of the ingredients one by one, making sure each is thoroughly blended before adding the next one. Stop the blender and push the pâté down toward the blades every now and then to assure thorough blending. if the pâté seems a bit dry, add a small amount of sherry or cognac (1 teaspoon). If you don't use alcohol, add a bit of water or chicken stock. The pâté should hold together nicely. You don't want it to be liquid. Fold in some pistachio nuts or chopped walnuts to add texture. Put the pâté in a clay crock, a clean jar or a bowl and cover tightly. Refrigerate and keep cool for at least 2 hours. It will become firmer as it cools. Serve on whole-grain bread cut into 1- by 1-inch squares or spread on lettuce leaves. (If you don't have a blender, use a fork or potato masher.)

COTTAGE-ROQUEFORT FILLING
(Makes about 1 cup. Keep refrigerated.)
⅛ pound cottage cheese
dash of Worcestershire sauce

⅛ pound Roquefort cheese
softened sweet butter (amount varies)

Using a fork, blend the cottage and Roquefort cheese. Add the Worcestershire sauce, and gradually add some sweet butter until the mixture becomes a slightly thick paste. Don't overdo the butter; it's merely there to hold the cheese together. You can add other seasonings to suit your taste. This mixture can be used to fill celery or mushroom caps, or can simply be rolled up in a lettuce leaf. (It is also a good spread for broiled chicken.)

TUNA-ONION FILLING

(This will fill a few dozen mushroom caps. Refrigerate.)
1 can water-packed tuna (Better to use freshly broiled tuna.)
1–2 tablespoons finely minced onion
1 tablespoon unsalted butter, softened
¼ cup ricotta cheese

Mix all the ingredients well and pile high on mushroom caps which have been washed and dried. Can be used as a filling for other vegetables as well.

VEGGIES-ON-A-STICK

For an easy-to-carry-around snack, marinate your favorite vegetables (raw and cut into 1″ squares) in a vinaigrette mixture. Then spear a variety on wooden skewers.

Other small snacks can be prepared from: broiled chicken drummettes (the meaty part of the wing) with curry powder or mustard; small meatballs, from a variety of meats that you grind at home and grill (we often grind liver, heart and beef together, adding some wheat germ to help them hold together).

Deviled eggs are prepared easily beforehand and can be stuffed not only by combining the egg yolk and mayonnaise mixture, but also by adding avocado, spices and other ground or grated vegetables or even fish or chicken (finely shredded).

Snack foods can be prepared with your regular meals and stored to be enjoyed later. Of course, raw foods, dairy products and fresh vegetable juices always make good, quick snacks.

FOOD
SUPPLEMENTS

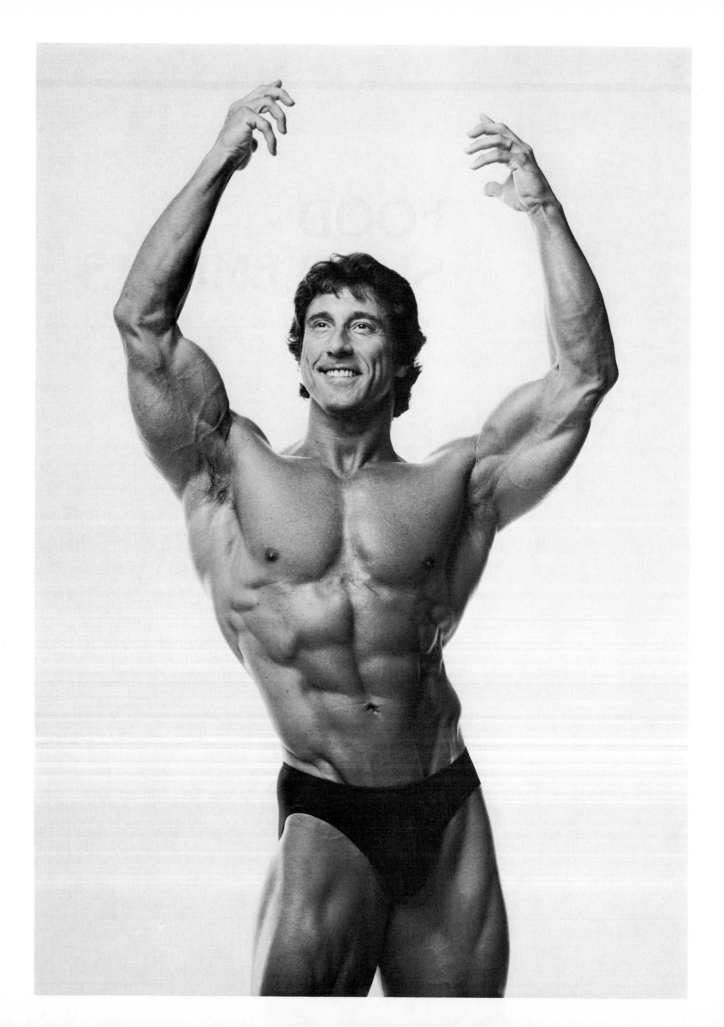

We all differ in our genetic makeup, hormone production, metabolic efficiency and nutritional requirements. Just because you may have discovered that a certain type of diet is best for you does not mean that this is the best type of diet for everyone. Some people are vitamin dependent. Their need for B vitamins, for example, may be 1,000 times the daily amount required by most people. If they do not receive this amount they may develop symptoms of a vitamin-deficiency disease. Supernutrition emphasizes the supplying of optimum nutrition to each cell in the body for the best possible health and resistance to disease.

Too often vitamins and minerals are lost in the process of food preparation. When you cut vegetables and fruits they are exposed to air and begin losing nutrients. That is why preparing your foods as close as possible to the time when you eat is advisable. If you peel foods and discard the peeling, you lose valuable nutrients that way, too. This is particularly true of soft-skinned foods like peaches, apples, potatoes, and so on. When you cook the food and it comes in contact with a combination of water, oxygen and heat, even more nutrients are lost. In fact, you could end up with just a lot of overseasoned, broken-down fiber instead of the nutritious food that you started out with. Avoid cooking on high heat, and steam foods instead of boiling them for a long time at high temperatures. Give your teeth something to chew! If we were meant to overcook everything until it fell apart and turned soft and mushy, we would only need gums! Most vitamins and minerals are stable during cooking at mild temperatures, but when the temperature is high—watch out.

Vitamin A is destroyed when over-oxygenated by frying in rancid oils or fats (vitamin A is fat soluble); however it is fairly stable in mild cooking. Most vegetables and fruits contain vitamin A.

Vitamin C is lost at room temperature through oxidation, so foods containing it should be kept cool. Cook over very low heat without water, if possible.

Vitamin D is stable in cooking, storing and oxidation.

Vitamin E can become rancid easily, but it is stable in cooking and with oxygenation.

Vitamin B complex varies in its stability depending on the individual vitamin. Thiamin (B_1) is very susceptible to being destroyed by heat, oxygen and alkaline substances like baking soda. (This is true of vitamin C as well). Toasting a piece of bread can destroy as much as 70% of the thiamin. Riboflavin (B_2) is found in milk and is very sensitive to slight increases as the temperature rises. It is stable in heat, however. Niacin (B_3) is water soluble but is generally the most stable of the B vitamins. Pyridoxine (B_6) is sensitive to heat, light and alkalinity in some foods, and it is usually lost in the refining process. Vitamin B_{12} can be destroyed in boiled milk, but it is stable under most conditions. The remainder of the B vitamin group is not affected by normal cooking; however, it is true that most of the B vitamins can be destroyed by alkaline conditions (using soda).

As many of your nutritional needs as possible should be met by the foods you eat; but since cooking destroys so many nutrients and eating the right foods isn't always possible, you may want to take vitamin, mineral, enzyme and/or protein supplements.

We usually take the following vitamin supplements daily:

vitamin A—10,000 i.u.
vitamin E—800 i.u.
niacidimide—50 mg
choline—1000 mg
folic acid, biotin, 100 mcg each
bioflavnoids—1000 mg
vitamin D—400 i.u.
vitamin B_1, B_2, B_6, PABA, niacin—
   50 mg each
calcium panothenate—200 mg
inositol—250 mg
vitamin C—3000 mg
B-15, rutin—100 mg each

We consider this a good maintenance program and often take two to three times these amounts when we want to look our very best.

Nutritional scientists have found special functions for Vitamin C and some of the B vitamins. Lack of thiamine (B_1) can affect your memory, appetite, moods and concentration. Niacin has been used for its fat-lowering properties because it can lower cholesterol levels in the blood. It is a strong vasodilator and when taken in higher amounts than you are used to will result in a flushing of the skin. In very high dosages, it is used by orthomolecular physicians to treat people with coronary disease, schizophrenia, allergies, senility and arthritis. Vitamin B_6 is needed by the body to make fifty different enzymes, must be present to metabolize all the amino acids and is necessary to maintain a stable immunologic system. In higher doses it works with vitamin C as a diuretic, has been used to combat premenstrual tensions, and to relieve tingling and numbness in the hands, leg cramps and arthritis. Vitamin B_{12} has been used to treat pernicious anemia, poor concentration, hallucinations, agitation and depression. Pantothenic acid along with vitamin C works directly on the adrenal glands to relieve stress. Individual requirements vary greatly.

We also take the following minerals:

calcium (from lactate, gluconate and citrate)—800 mg
phosphorous and magnesium (from oxide)—400 mg
iodine—225 mcg
selenium—300 mcg
iron, zinc and manganese—30 mg each
trace minerals—15 mg total
potassium—50 mg

Calcium can be lost by high temperatures, water and by oxidation. Chlorine and fluorine are destroyed by high temperatures. Iron, which gives us pep by carrying oxygen through the blood, is destroyed by water and oxidation. Phosphorus and magnesium (a natural laxative) can both be destroyed by water and high heat. Potassium, manganese (works with your nervous system and helps improve your memory), silicon (a blood builder) and sodium (a blood purifier) are all destroyed or leached by water. Iodine and sulphur (needed by the nervous system, brain, skin, hair and nails) are destroyed by oxidation and high temperatures.

We suggest that you take vitamins and minerals when you eat, and take them slowly. Vitamins enclosed in gelatin capsules are rapidly dissolved in your stomach and consequently reach the blood stream quickly. Vitamins and minerals compressed into a pill and held together with bulky, inert materials or binders should never be used. Unless a time-release vitamin is in a gelatin capsule, there is no guarantee that it will dissolve enough in your stomach to be absorbed. Be sure to hold gelatin capsules in your mouth 30 seconds before swallowing with a liquid, so your saliva softens the capsule. Never take vitamins containing sugar or preservatives.

If you want to build more solid muscle, you should consider taking a protein supplement. Our favorite is milk and egg protein. From our experience, liquid protein made from collagen, which is derived from connective tissue of cattle, is not as effective. Glandular protein powders are made from animal's internal organs (i.e., liver, heart, spleen); but they do not taste good and do not supply calcium, as a milk/egg protein does. Protein powders can be mixed with food, like yogurt or cottage cheese, or can be sipped in a drink mixture of milk or cream and water. Never gulp down protein drinks, sip them slowly.

Hydrochloric acid and digestive enzymes are present in your stomach to break down protein into amino acids. Protein digestants are often used when a lot of protein is being consumed. We take these digestants daily when our protein intake is high:

betaine hcl.—800 mg
pepsin—300 mg
glutamic acid hcl.—600 mg

The papain in papaya and the bromeline in pineapple also work to aid protein digestion.

If you don't like the idea of opening ten or more vitamin bottles every day, you may want to take a multiple vitamin/mineral. We suggest you take one that has all the nutrients we described along with extra vitamin C and vitamin E. Natural foods, like dessicated liver, torula and brewers yeast, are good sources of B vitamins, iron and amino acids. Lecithin (the natural fat emulsifier found in eggs and soybeans) is a good natural source of phosphorous, choline and inositol and is good for the skin and hair.

Your way of eating should neither interfere with your enjoyment of dining out with friends nor make you feel self-conscious at the dinner table at home. Adding nutritional supplements to your diet can be a way of taking the worry out of whether or not you are getting proper nutrition.

MAKING THE BEST CHOICES IN YOUR DIET

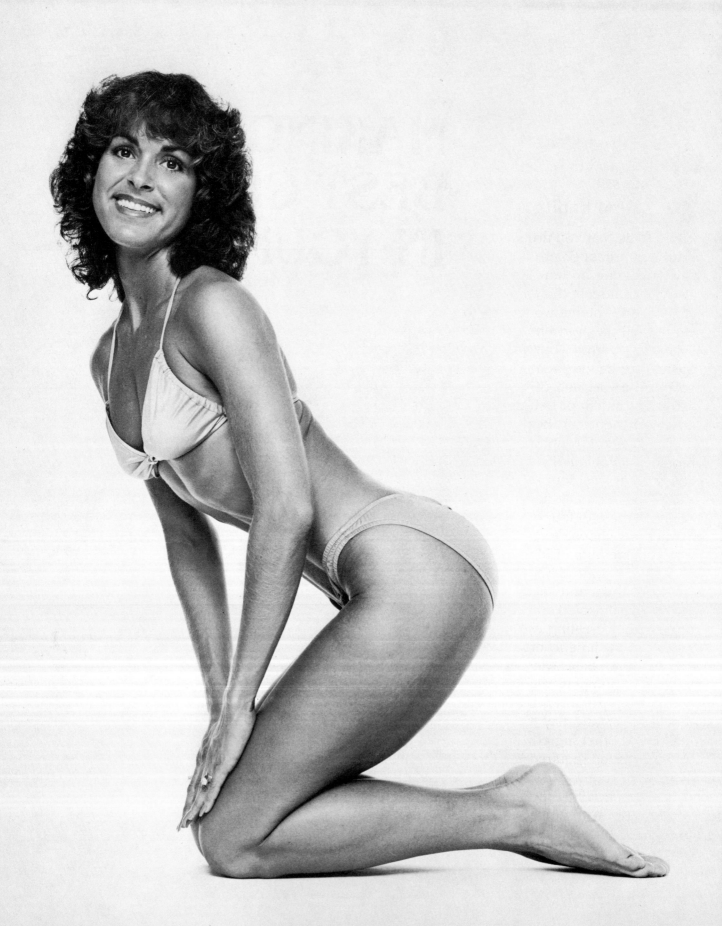

Your Eating Habits

If the foods that you are eating are natural and healthy, what about your eating habits? Are they natural and healthy too? These habits have a bearing on how food will be used by your body. You should always eat at least three meals a day. This keeps your digestive and elimination systems working regularly. Your body will adapt to this easily within a short time. Eating regular meals and refraining from overeating permit your system to assimilate more and leave less waste. Overeating is another habit that can be broken by regular, balanced meals and, if necessary, small snacks between breakfast and a late lunch, or between an early lunch and dinner. Snacks that are timed right can help prevent overeating. Get into the habit of drinking water throughout the day and at bedtime. You need this for proper functioning of your organs, as well as for healthy-looking skin. You need at least four extra glasses of plain water in addition to that which you normally have in your diet—assuming that you already drink in excess of four or five glasses a day.

What you choose to eat can also be the result of habit rather than wise consideration. Did you know that the weather has a strong effect on you? On warm days you should eat differently than on cold days. Eat more fruits and salads on those hot summer days. These foods are quickly digested and do not cause the body to overwork and "fire up," thereby creating excess body heat. Starches, proteins and fats require more time to digest, so are better choices for cold weather. Nature knows best. Winter vegetables tend to be more starchy—like yams and pumpkin. Summer foods, such as melons and summer squashes, are lighter. Don't judge a food by its temperature to the touch. Ice cream may feel cold, but as your body digests the heavy cream and other ingredients, it becomes a heat-producing food. The more digestion required, the more heat will be produced.

Chewing your foods improperly is a poor habit. Starches need to be chewed especially well to mix with the saliva and digestive juices in your mouth. With crunchy starches, like carrots, it is easier to chew them well, but often soft starches such as potatoes are swallowed long before they have had a chance to mix well with the saliva. Pay particular attention to chewing these softer starches. You may not be getting all the nutrients you had hoped to from your foods, and digestive problems could occur later. Raw foods need to be chewed thoroughly to break down the cell walls.

A very bad habit you can adopt at an early age is salting your food. Table salt is not necessary in your diet. Get rid of it. When you are eating plenty of natural foods, you will get all the salt you need. If you wish to flavor your foods use powdered forms of vegetables which have a higher content of natural sodium. These powdered concentrates can be found in most health food stores. Salts are found in larger amounts in the peelings and outer parts of fruits and vegetables. Eat more of these types of foods instead of adding salt. For this reason we eat very little of the inside of the potato, because it has too much starch for our needs. We do eat the skins and about ½ to ¼ inch of the part found just under the skin, so that we get more minerals and less of the starch. Excess salt in your diet can cause water retention in your body and thus a puffy, swollen look and weight gain. This water retention interferes with the passing of toxins from your system.

Slow down when you eat. Don't rush. Enjoy your food. When you eat . . . eat. Watching TV or reading while eating is a distraction and can lead to overeating. Instead, try to savor every bite and delight in the food's attractive appearance and texture. As we have stressed throughout, eat your largest meal early in the day. Food eaten later in the evening can more easily turn into fat on your waist, hips or upper arms.

Also, arguing at mealtime or playing loud music with a fast-beating rhythm can cause stomach and digestion problems. If you suffer an emotional upset right before a meal, it is probably better to skip the meal until a time when you are in a better state of mind and body, and can relax first before eating. We have heard of people who like to sit down for a quiet ten minutes before each meal. This sounds like a good practice if you tend to be under pressure or be frequently vulnerable to tension-producing situations.

You should not get in the habit of giving up your new way of eating because you may have "cheated" a bit at one time. If you happen to slip up, return to your healthful way of eating right away. Starving and punishing yourself seldom works. Invariably it will only push you deeper into a pattern of indulging yourself, then feeling guilty about what you have done, and then starving yourself so that you lose all hope of attaining your goal and start the cycle all over again. Break the cycle before it takes hold. Realize that on occasion you may slip up, but return immediately to your healthful eating ways.

Thinking positively about yourself and about your goals is a most effective approach. Seeing yourself as you know you are and as being capable of success can keep you moving forward. When you are happy and feeling positive about yourself, your body and mind work together better. If you ever find yourself having "down" thoughts or in a foul mood, bring yourself out of the dumps by thinking about positive, happy things. Only you can do this for yourself. When you try, you'll see it's impossible to feel bad when thinking cheerful and "up" thoughts.

Raw Food in Your Diet

Eating raw food makes more vitamins and minerals available to your body. Raw food demands more vigorous digestion, since you need to break down the cell walls to make assimilation easier. Vigorous physical activity on a regular basis, such as the exercises you are doing in this program, help to improve the digestive process.

Many vitamins are very sensitive to heat and are destroyed by cooking. Vitamin C is one of them. Eating fruits high in Vitamin C in their fresh, natural, raw state will give you more of the nutrients you are seeking. The same is true of juice. Processed and concentrated juice in cans or bottles have lost much of their vitamin and mineral content. Foods in their raw state are different from the same foods cooked. Raw foods are known to contain large amounts of hidden nutrients that cannot be produced and added by man. These can only be obtained by eating food in its natural, raw condition. When you eat raw foods, chew them well. Starches and sugars begin digesting in your mouth, so unless the cell walls are broken down here, digestion may take longer. If your digestive system is not ready for the vigorous digesting of raw foods and for handling great amounts of bulk in the system, and your teeth are weaker from following a diet of soft-cooked, over-processed foods, you should begin adding raw foods to your diet in liquid form. This means vegetables and fruits pureed and juiced. Blending, pureeing and juicing all aid your digestive system by breaking down the cellulose and making the nutrients locked inside the food more available for assimilation. Your body gets the benefits with less work. Raw, fresh juices and pureed foods need to be eaten as soon as they are prepared, because cutting food exposes it to air and valuable nutrients are lost if the food is left standing for too long. When preparing raw foods by any of these methods, remember that juices and purees are more concentrated and shouldn't be eaten in large quantities. Some vegetables like beets, watercress, radishes and parsley are very strong in taste and potent in effect and should be mixed or diluted with other juices that are not as powerful—such as celery, spinach, carrot, tomato and cucumber as well as with mineral water. Try to include some raw foods in your diet each day. If you feel you would benefit from eating more raw foods, you might try a day when you eat a majority of your meals this way. Raw foods contain the essence of life.

Digestion

All foods are not digested in the same way. Each type of food requires its own method of digestion and its own digestive juices. When you chew, digestive juices begin secreting in the stomach and saliva is secreted in the mouth. Sometimes we don't even need to chew to start the juices flowing. We've all experienced this when we see someone eating a lemon or smell a dill pickle! Sugars are absorbed to some extent in your mouth, but with other foods there is actually very little absorption taking place there. Food entering your stomach causes peristalsis to begin. This action carries the food through your intestines and on to being eliminated. The peristaltic action is much faster during meals than between meals. Some absorption occurs in your stomach but it mainly takes place in your small intestines. The function of your large intestines is primarily elimination. Through all these processes the digestive secretions break down the food that you eat. Saliva digests starchy foods; gastric juices secreted in the stomach digest proteins; bile secreted by your liver digests fats; and pancreatic juices digest both fats and starches. Whatever is left is taken care of by the intestines. Intestinal juices digest all foods.

There are many other factors that stimulate digestion. Your attitude is one of them, the temperature of your foods is another and the order in which you eat your foods also affects when they will be digested.

After you have eaten, wait a significant amount of time before you engage in any physical activity. Try to time your meals so you will be able to lie down and relax afterward.

Acidity and Alkalinity

You may have heard about acid-producing foods and alkaline-producing foods. The body functions better when it is in an alkaline, or close to neutral, condition. This is not always possible, especially with all the acid-producing meat in our diet. A meatless diet does bring your body to an alkaline state; but, at the same time, you must know which foods will supply the right amount of protein to nourish and repair the body's tissues. If you balance the acid-producing foods with the alkaline-producing foods you will stay closer to an alkaline state. Generally your body adjusts itself to the foods that you eat, but it can happen that a diet that is too acidic can be disease-producing; you may suffer from such disorders as diarrhea or respiratory problems. Good health usually exists in conjunction with an alkaline or neutral system, and some people only eat one type of food at a time to achieve this balance. We prefer variety and so don't recommend this kind of restricted diet.

Many foods have an acid taste but are actually alkaline producing. Tomatoes, onions, grapefruit, oranges, limes and berries are all alkaline producing but taste acidic. Generally, proteins and starchy foods are acid producing. If you would like to find out more about the acidity and alkalinity of the foods you are eating, get a book at your health food store which goes into greater detail about these foods. One of the reasons that we recommend drinking sparkling mineral water with most of your meals, especially when they are extremely high in protein, is that it aids both in deacidifying your stomach and in digesting your food.

Macronutrients

PROTEIN

Assimilability is a measure of the extent to which a protein is absorbed in the body. The proteins most easily used, that is, those highest in assimilability, are eggs and dairy products—90 to 95 percent assimilable; fish, poultry and meats—approximately 80 percent assimilable; and vegetable proteins, such as brewers yeast and soybeans—about 50 percent assimilable. It makes sense to depend for at least some of your protein on the foods with the highest assimilability.

Protein foods comprise the largest part of our diet. We prefer to eat chicken, fresh fish, eggs and dairy products as our sources of protein. If you are not a strict vegetarian, you'll want to stick to these choices. These foods are higher in protein and, with the exception of cheese, lower in fats. Red meats, such as beef, pork and lamb contain more fat. Even the leanest cuts are still about 30 to 40 percent fat. Red meat works well in the diet for those who want to put on body weight. You'll probably notice that when you begin eating fish, chicken and eggs for your protein, you'll feel lighter and will drop excess body fat. At some markets you can purchase grain-fed chickens which were not fed chemicals or hormones. We choose these because they taste more flavorful to us.

By keeping a record of our protein intake we have found 1 to 2 grams of protein per pound of body weight is necessary for building muscle and approximately ½ to ¾ gram of protein per pound of body weight is necessary for maintaining muscle size and tone. By keeping your careful records you will be able to tell if these amounts vary for your body.

Protein is composed of amino acids. Eighteen different amino acids should be present in our food. Of these, there are eight that must be supplied by the foods we eat because the body can't make them. They are valine, lysine, threonine, leucine, isoleucine, tryptophan, phenylalanine, and methionine. These are called the essential amino acids. If these amino acids are not supplied in our diet the body can't build complete protein in the form of muscle. The body can only use the L-form of the amino acid.

Certain amino acids have special properties when taken in larger amounts. Among the ones we use are:

Tryptophan can be used to help induce sleep when taken in doses of 1 to 2 grams on a relatively empty stomach.

Glutamine removes toxic waste from the brain and helps maintain cerebral tissues. A teaspoon of glutamine can help increase attention, persistence and performance of repetitive tasks.

Methionine is a sulphur containing amino acid, acts as a lipotropic agent or fat carrier in the bloodstream and, along with choline and inositol, prevents fat from adhering to the walls of the blood vessels.

Tyrosine helps stabilize blood sugar levels when taken after meals.

Cystine is needed for healthy hair and skin and is believed to retard aging.

CARBOHYDRATES

Choosing foods that are lower in carbohydrates and fats will enable you to become leaner than before. Use your food almanac to check the carbohydrate value of foods. The total number of carbohydrates that you allow yourself per day will depend on how well your body handles the different carbohydrates, how active you are and other factors, like your size and the condition of your health. You can determine how many carbohydrates you use daily by your level of activity. If you are not very active you may need only 40 to 80 grams daily. If you are moderately active you may need only 80 to 150 grams daily. If you are very active you may need 150 to 250 grams daily. This is only a rough guide to your carbohydrate level, and these amounts vary widely among individuals. Carbohydrates are necessary for the proper functioning of your organs, especially the brain. Don't ever eliminate them entirely for long periods of time.

Carbohydrates are of two types: sugars and starches. The best source of sugars are fruits that give you a rush of energy a few minutes after they are eaten. Starches take longer to break down and provide energy over a longer time (usually several hours). The best sources of starches are vegetables and whole-grain products.

An overabundance of refined and/or processed carbohydrates (sugar, white flour, "convenient" highly processed foods) or too much alcohol, coffee, tea, cola drinks and tobacco can cause hypoglycemia or low blood sugar. Complex carbohydrates can eliminate low blood sugar symptoms because they require 4 or more hours to digest and provide a more constant flow of glucose to the body than do the more quickly absorbed refined and processed simple sugars. Some symptoms of hypoglycemia are: loss of memory, lack of concentration, emotional instability, impatience, irritability, depression, abnormal sensitivity to light, fatigue, weakness, insomnia, dizziness and fainting spells, headaches, muscle and joint pains. These symptoms usually occur ½ to 2 hours after eating. From personal experiments, we have found that ½ to 1 gram of carbohydrate per pound of body weight will provide high energy and a more congenial disposition. Zero to ¼ gram of carbohydrate per pound of body weight will provide more fat loss (because low carbohydrate intake forces the body to mobilize its stored fat) but less energy for workouts. Our brains use up to 70 percent of the carbohydrates that we consume.

FATS
Fats are of two kinds: saturated—from animal, dairy and egg sources (lard, butter, cream, egg yolks); and unsaturated—from vegetable sources (lecithin, wheat germ oil, safflower oil, corn oil, etc.). Your body needs slightly more saturated than unsaturated fats. Too much unsaturated fat could cause a vitamin E deficiency.

Fats are needed in the body for healthy hair, skin and internal organs and mucous membrane formation. Fats also help a person on a diet not to feel hungry because they take longer to digest and empty out of the stomach more slowly. To lose weight we have found the most success when less than 6 calories per pound of body weight from fat sources is consumed daily; however, this amount varies widely between individuals.

Micronutrients

Micronutrients refers to vitamins and minerals; these nutrients need to be present in the body in smaller amounts, usually milligrams or even micrograms (one millionth of a gram). Vitamins are essential substances which can't be made in the body. They are used to form enzymes which catalyze reactions in the body. Each enzyme is a protein, made up of hundreds of amino acids (building blocks of protein) and often vitamins, combined in the right way. Minerals are substances present in the body's cells and needed by them in their construction and function.

Vitamins are of two kinds: water soluble (B and C complex) and fat soluable (A, D, and E). Water-soluble vitamins pass through and out of the body in four to six hours, so they should be taken more often than fat-soluble vitamins, which the body can store. Minerals are water soluble and, as with vitamins, the optimal amounts vary from person to person. It is preferable to obtain the majority of the vitamin and minerals that we need from our foods.

The B complex vitamins consist of at least 10 known types: B_1, B_2, niacin or niacidamide, B_6, B_{12}, biotin, folic acid, PABA, panothenic acid, and B_{15}. The B complex vitamins are essential for proper protein, carbohydrate and fat metabolism and are needed for a healthy nervous system; they also keep your appetite and digestion normal. Co-vitamins, choline and inositol, the lipotropic agents, act as fat emulsifiers in the bloodstream and assist in preventing fats from adhering to the blood vessel walls. Choline is needed by the body to make acetylcholine which is needed at nerve synapses for the transmission of nerve impulses and muscle contraction. When acetylcholine is low, the body's muscles won't contract properly.

Vitamin C and bioflavnoids and rutin form the C complex, an anti-oxidant, which helps protect the body from environmental pollution, builds resistance to infection, assists in the formation of collagen, the intercellular connective tissue, helps in the healing of wounds and fractures, aids in strengthening capillaries, bones and gums and assists in the proper utilization of iron. Bioflavnoids and rutin aid in the body's utilization of vitamin C.

Vitamins A, D and E are fat-soluble vitamins, and the body can store them. Vitamin A is essential for night vision, keeps linings of your nose, throat and digestive system healthy and improves skin texture. Vitamin D promotes normal growth of bones and teeth. It is possible to build up too much vitamins A and D if very large doses are taken over a period of several months. Harmful side effects from very high dosage of vitamin E are not evident, as in the case vitamins A and D. As an anti-oxidant, vitamin E is the most important in protecting the body against damaging substances, formed when oxygen reacts directly with unsaturated fatty acids. It is thought to be a means of preventing premature aging, as well as being beneficial to the heart, reproductive, and circulatory systems of the body.

Minerals should come from our diet as much as possible. When minerals are obtained from food, they are "chelated" or bound to organic molecules from which they slowly release in the body. The major minerals are: calcium—helps develop and maintain strong teeth and bones, assists muscle action, heart and nerve function and blood clotting and promotes a feeling of calmness; phosphorous—works with calcium in muscle contraction and nerve response; magnesium—aids in nerve relaxation, construction of body protein and reduction of blood pressure; iron—carries oxygen to the cells after it combines with protein to form hemoglobin; iodine—needed in small amounts (micrograms) by the body, it functions with the thyroid gland to regulate body metabolism, and mental and physical development; potassium—helps prevent muscle cramping and weakness, fatigue and indifference.

Trace minerals are needed in small amounts and are vital factors in maintaining physiological processes (chlorine, chromium, copper, fluorine, manganese, selenium, sodium, vanadium and zinc). Of special importance are manganese (aids in fat utilization and activates numerous enzyme systems) and selenium (an anti-oxidant which helps protect the body from environmental pollution and premature aging). Selenium has also been found to have anabolic properties. Chromium is essential for the body to utilize sugar properly and reacts with protein and stimulates several enzyme systems. Zinc helps the body use lactic acid developed during exercise (excess lactic acid is responsible for muscular soreness) and is essential for the synthesis of protein and the action of over thirty enzymes. Deficiency of zinc affects smell, taste and appetite and may cause lethargy. A high phosphorous diet (high in red meat) may produce zinc deficiency. Drinking water high in copper or lead should be avoided, since it can be poisonous to your system in some amounts.

Certain non-chelated minerals like iron and zinc can destroy vitamin E and selenium. To prevent this we take vitamin E and selenium in the morning and iron and zinc later in the day.

BODY PART INDEX